The Pharmacist's Secrets

Drugs, lies and money

Robert Gosstray

MIDLIFEXPRESS ePUBLISHING
TASMANIA
© 2014

MIDLIFEXPRESS
PUBLISHED BY MIDLIFEXPRESS EPUBLISHING
MIDLIFEXPRESS.COM
MIDLIFEX@MIDLIFEXPRESS.COM
TASMANIA, AUSTRALIA

COPYRIGHT © ROBERT GOSSTRAY

ALL RIGHTS RESERVED. NO PART OF THIS PRODUCT MAY BE REPRODUCED, SCANNED, OR DISTRIBUTED IN ANY PRINTED OR ELECTRONIC FORM WITHOUT PERMISSION.

THIS MATERIAL HAS PREVIOUSLY APPEARED IN MIDLIFEXPRESS

PRINT ISBN: 1502723093

The Legal Stuff

This book is designed to provide helpful information and suggestions on the subjects herein. Its author(s) and publisher are not offering professional advice of any kind, including psychological, legal, financial or medical.

The publisher and author(s) bear no responsibility for any specific health or allergy needs that may require medical supervision and are not liable for any damages or negative consequences from any treatment, action, application or preparation, to any person reading or following information in this book.

The content of each article or chapter is the opinion of its author, and not necessarily that of the publisher. No warranties or guarantees are expressed or implied by the publisher's choice to include any of the content in this volume.

Neither the publisher nor the individual author shall be liable for any physical, psychological, emotional, financial, or commercial damages, including, but not limited to, special, incidental, consequential or other damages.

References are provided for information purposes only and do not constitute endorsement of the website or other sources.

From the Author

My 50 odd (some say 'very odd') years in pharmacy have convinced me we have taken a wrong turn in our reliance on quick-fix drugs for our modern ailments. My father and grandfather were both pharmacists, so that pharmaceutical influence has extended from about 1900 to the present day. I still have a love and reverence for the art of compounding extemporaneous medicines, a practice that has almost completely disappeared. I realise there were no magic cures then, but now also realise there are still no magic cures, despite what medical orthodoxy and monolithic drug companies would have you believe. The following articles, based on my memory and opinions, describe aspects of my career and reflect on some of the frightening modern-day drug treatments we have been subjected to.

Robert Gosstray 2014

Table of Contents

DRUGS
Life: Want a Drug With That?	8
Legal Addiction	10
The War on Drugs	12
Injecting Fear - The War on Drugs	14
Addicts I Have Known	16
All drugged up and nowhere to go	21
Grannies, Drugs and Money	23

CONTRACEPTION
To Be Or Not To Be - That is the QES-tion?	25
You Wouldn't Conceive of It	27
Not in My Backyard	29
Pill - Oh Talk	30

CANCER
Why we need a new attitude to cancer	32
Mini health report: The cancers that won't kill you	34
Why Cannabis should be used in cancer treatments	35

HEALTH
Why our food is making us sick	37
Human health sniffles towards Bethlehem	38
Why the diet industry is a big fat rip off	40
Save on health products and suck on a tree instead	42
A holistic health system is the way forward	44

PHARMACEUTICALS
Why off labelling drug prescription is off its head	47
How to be the world's most inept drug pusher	49
Rotigotine: Another drug with weird and wonderful side effects	51
Sighed Effects - What drugs really do to you	52
Why modern medicine is failing us all	55
Poppin pills ain't curin' ills	57
Why we crumble as we age and how modern medicine makes it worse	61
How our toxic environment is playing havoc with our children's health	63

THE GOLDEN AGE
From Shaman to Pharman': Pharmacy's lost heritage	65
A modern alchemist recalls the golden years of pharmacy	68
Vale the pharmacy of old	70
The aromatic heaven of the pharmacy of old	72
Why I'm uneasy about our magic fix society	75
Peak advertising of harmful products is here	78

DRUGS

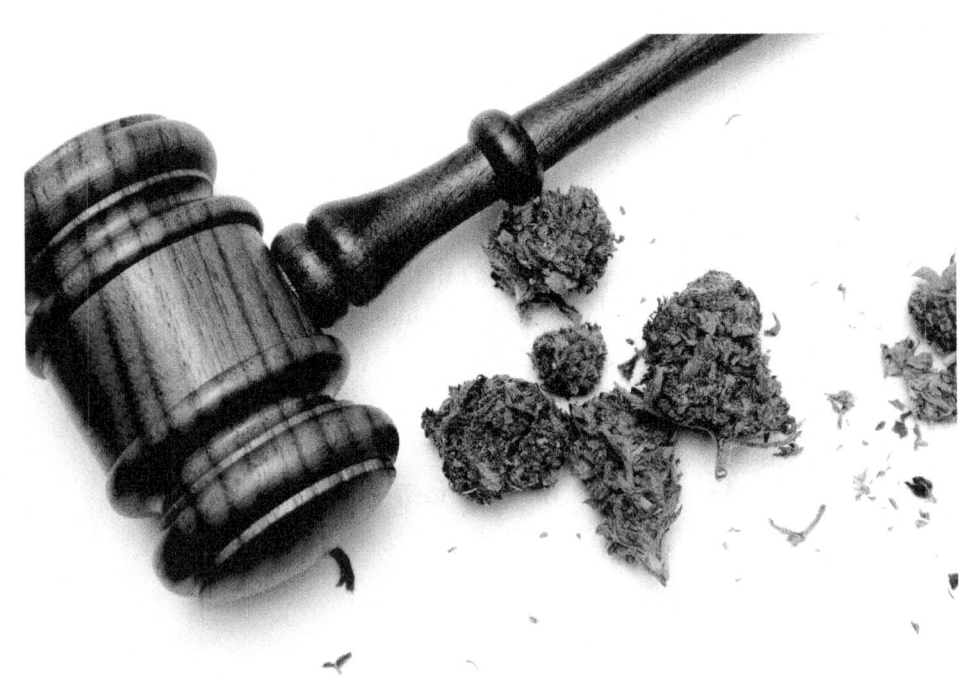

Life:Want a Drug With That?

As a pharmacist, my experience with providing medical treatments lasted for over fifty years. Over this time, I have become disillusioned and cynical about our modern drug-taking culture.

Historically, our present day drugs mostly derived from naturally occurring plant and animal compounds. These had been used for hundreds of years, throughout the world, and had some degree of usefulness in relieving pain, improving mood, treating infections, inducing sleep and alleviating other benign disorders. They were ineffective treating the major disorders such as heart disease, cancer, arthritis, lung disease and severe mental illness.

The sorry story is that all the modern drugs we use to treat these major disorders are nearly as useless; moreover, they have much more severe side-effects. The path we have taken is for everyone to seek out and demand perfect health. We want to live forever and so that's what the modern medical system tries to provide. Doctors, researchers and drug companies have formed an unwritten and unholy alliance hell-bent on providing an instant miracle - drug cure for every conceivable ailment.

A case in point is the Hormone Replacement Therapy (HRT) industry. It's an ongoing, wretched saga spanning decades. Menopause has somehow come to be seen by doctors and their female patients as a "disorder". However, menopause is a normal life condition that midlife women have survived quite well for millennia, yet many women began to demand a "treatment" for its symptoms.

The medical and drug industries were happy to provide hormones derived from horse serum (mares of course) for their flushed clients. Serious side effects of HRT - such as blood clots - were ignored or downplayed. There is an army of "experts" employed by each drug company to make sure their products are viewed in a favourable way (similar to the 'experts' employed by the tobacco companies and the breweries). It's time to question the need for drugs in many instances and to take a more philosophical view of life's physical stages.

I am appalled by the direction in which modern medicine is heading. I've been retired from pharmacy for almost two years now and I still read up on the latest horrors. The Western world is suffering epidemics of obesity, diabetes, heart disease, cancers, depression and arthritis. Our children are increasingly unhealthy and many are born with ADHD, autism, dystrophies and other serious conditions. People demand instant fixes for all these things, so that's what they get.

Dabigatran is a new drug to replace Warfarin as a blood thinner. Warfarin is cheap but effective - with the disadvantage of requiring frequent blood tests. Dabigatran costs an arm and a leg (not literally), is equally effective BUT has been found to sometimes cause fatal hemorrhage. AND - there is no antidote. Great work, fellas.

The monoclonal antibodies are now sweeping the world and - if you are ordered a drug with a funny name ending in 'mab' - run for your life. These have been developed at great cost (to everyone) to treat the modern-day epidemics of so-called 'auto-immune' diseases - cancers, arthritis and other problems that can't be explained. Using gene therapies and experimental mice, chickens and cows, the MABS are created and then spliced onto human antibodies. Costing thousands of dollars with each treatment, they are then used as immune-suppressants, the theory being they will prevent human rogue antibodies from causing disease.

Great theory, but stuffing around with the very complex human immune system is just stupid. All kinds of side effects occur - opportunistic infections of course - which can be fatal, as well as far-reaching reactions body-wide.

I actually laughed out loud at a recent report on one of the latest MABS, which solemnly stated that one side-effect was "homicidal Ideation" and another one was "suicidal Ideation" – that is, you thought killing yourself or someone else was a good idea.

Our medical system needs to acknowledge that we are all a collection of cells (called 'life'); some good and healthy, others defective. Medicine needs to focus on prevention (improving environmental factors) rather than treating modern-day 'life-style' disorders with dangerous, expensive and mostly useless drugs.

Legal Addiction

I have the greatest respect for the clever, sometimes brilliant, concerned and compassionate doctors and surgeons in our system, but they are faced with impossible tasks and demands. You only have to read the daily papers to notice the multi-page ads for grog (the worst addiction - particularly with young people) and drugs (dished out on special—two for the price of one, we will not be beaten on price etc.).

Huge and impersonal drug warehouses cater for our society's obsession and craving for the good life. There are drugs for anxiety, gut relief, detox, sleep-aids, wake-up aids, "miracle" arthritis, psoriasis and baldness cures, weird supplements from krill (have you ever seen a nervous or anxious whale?), memory tonics, weight-loss and weight gain supplements, libido stimulants for men and women, stress relief, menopause relief and a multitude of vitamins, minerals and herbs all guaranteed to make you live forever (but if you die, you get your money cheerfully refunded at the funeral).

These are just the over-the-counter items. Also advertised are cheap prescription items With such promotion, along with the promotion of gambling, drinking and junk food, is it any wonder western societies are addicted, frenzied, stressed, fearful and unhealthy.

In the last few years of my working life, I was staggered by the extent of legal addictions occurring (and encouraged). People were becoming hooked on Ventolin spray, codeine containing preparations (Mersyndol, Nurofen Plus, various cough mixtures, Panadeine products), sleeping pills (Dozile, Restavit, Stilnox) and sedating anti-histamines. There was also a marked rise in the use of prescription narcotics—Oxynorm, Oxycontin, MS Contin and others- I think doctors had just given up and ordered these for anyone who had a sore back.

Another problem was the supply of pseudo-ephedrine. This drug is highly effective as a decongestant for use in respiratory tract infections, and for clearing airways to the ear in aeroplane travel.

It can also be a precursor for the manufacture of amphetamines, so bikie gangs would send out "mules" to buy up as much legal pseudo-ephedrine as possible. The banning of amphetamines has led to police corruption, burglary, murder and super-rich gangsters and this stupid policy naturally led on to the virtual banning of pseudo-ephedrine. It has now been removed from most products and replaced with less effective decongestants (phenylephrine and phenylpropanolamine), which also have more side-effects. The pack sizes of pseudo-ephedrine were drastically reduced – this meant that the bikies' mules had to work harder and travel more.

The official directions for pharmacists was for us to closely question every purchaser, check whether their noses were dribbling and ask for ID. During my night-time shifts, you can imagine how many times I did this when a fat, balding bikie swinging a chain came in and pretended he was dying from a cold. I never knocked anybody back—

they all got what they wanted and everyone was happy (especially me when that chain didn't finish up wrapped around my neck).

I will finish off by reporting the latest lunacy in our "war on drugs". A scientific paper has just been published by a group of medical nongs, stating earnestly that marijuana use by the young causes anxiety attacks in later life. Nowhere was it suggested that perhaps it was anxiety that persuaded the young people to try marijuana in the first place. We are continuing to get it all back to front.

The War on Drugs

This is a personal recollection of my time trying to help drug addicts. When I first started as a pharmacist in the 1950's and 60's, every pharmacy supplied many addicts, but not with illicit street drugs. Our addicts were usually little old ladies - oppressed, poor and mired in dull suburban conformity. To escape the monotony and the pain, they became hooked on such things as Chloral Hydrate sleeping mixture, Senega and Ammonia cough mixture (which at that time contained Camphorated Tincture of Opium), Chlorodyne for diarrhoea (containing Morphine Tincture and chloroform), "Four Three-penn'ths" (a brilliant combination of laudanum, paregoric, aniseed and peppermint spirits). I loved the idea of "Four Three-penn'ths", which was developed in the UK and derived its name from charging threepence each for the four ingredients.

Of course, in Australia (and after decimal currency arrived) the price would be nothing like four threepences (one shilling). It was still cheap and was used by the desperate housewives of the time - for just about every known complaint - but its main value was its soothing and reassuring addictive properties. Barbiturate sleeping drugs were widely prescribed at the time. There were many varieties and they were very effective, very addictive and very damaging to livers and kidneys. However, supply and demand meant that the desperate housewives demanded and the compliant medicos supplied.

As pharmacists, we knew all our local addicts but, to me, it was all part of a broken social system. We and the doctors were the first 'drug pushers', bending under the assault of terrifying, wild-eyed and threatening suburban housewives in order to supply their habit. Of course, men had their addictions too, but generally confined them to grog, smokes, gambling, meat pies, the footy and Holden cars. However, when the amphetamines arrived, men were the biggest users, becoming hooked on dexamphetamine and methamphetamine, supplied in copious amounts by their friendly local doctors and pharmacists. My theory is that women blocked out their dull and oppressed lives with sedatives and legal opiates, while men were desperate to stay young, revved-up and dominating with stimulants.

Here follows a brief confession (of sorts). I have smoked 'pot' – not much, but quite relaxing and enjoyable (as were cigarettes) - and have used amphetamines. A few fellow students and I tried them a few times to help us cram for exams. I found them to be all right for increasing short-term confidence, but useless for any long-term value. In fact, they were detrimental as the false confidence faded quickly to be replaced by our usual air of befuddlement.

Despite anything I write here, I am not an advocate for any drug, legal or illegal. I have seen the damage done by both forms.

Back to the 50's and 60's (my favourite era - heavy sigh), the LOLS (little old ladies, not laugh out louds) were still pouring in seeking their nirvana in Relaxa Tabs and other sedatives. They were also hooked on Bex powders. Instead of supplying good old aspirin in tablet form (boring), the cunning manufacturers wrapped the prescribed dose in dinky little, origami-like, paper packages. This gave the aspirin an air of mystery and effectiveness, and was probably the initiator of the housewives' mantra: A nice cup of tea, a Bex and a good lie down.

This was fine as it made their lives a little more bearable, but our esteemed guardians of correctness in everything (while everything was about to become as incorrect as possible), virtually banned aspirin in this form due to occasional kidney problems. I still believe aspirin is one of the best drugs ever produced, when used sensibly, but the bad press from the "Bex Powder" scandals, allied to later reports of sporadic and minor bleeding from the stomach linings, virtually killed it off. It has now been replaced by Paracetamol (less effective and the major cause of overdose, poisoning and hospital admissions) and Ibuprofen (even less effective and implicated in serious side-effects).

Australia's futile "war on drugs" started at this time, following America's lead who had banned alcohol (prohibition in the 1930's) and marijuana in the 1940's (everyone should see the film "Reefer Madness" for a good laugh as wild-eyed, slavering youths smoking joints, descend into depravity by not saluting the American flag). These bans refuse to recognise the inherent addictive nature of many people, who need all sorts of weird things to get them through the day. One of our classic LOL addicts was actually hooked on "Mentos", the peppermint sweet. She would order them by the carton, often appearing with white, menthol dribble down her chin. Under our repressive and idiotic laws, she would be jailed as a "user" and me as a "menthol trafficker".

My next article will cover the late 1960's when we lurched into the aftermath of the Vietnam war, with street drugs (mainly heroin) reaching Australia. This is where the "Reefer Madness" mentality afflicted our politicians, church leaders, law makers and police with disastrous and continuing results.

Injecting Fear - The War on Drugs

Inspired by our lords, masters and fellow war criminals in Vietnam, we dutifully tagged along as American soldiers took to heroin in an effort to block out the horrible things they were forced to do. The Americans took their heroin habits back home, as did the Australians, and heroin flooded the streets in most Western cities. It took off really quickly here, mainly amongst disaffected, rebellious and poor young people. Our ever alert authorities acted quickly - that is, they panicked and banned all manufacture and imports of heroin in Australia. This was the first blow in the futile "War on Drugs", again following the lead set by the US.

I still had stocks of heroin powder stashed away in our Dangerous Drugs cupboard—not a security priority as it was an ancient, wooden box with a ply-wood door and a flimsy, token lock and key. Up until this complete ban, we still dispensed Heroin Linctus (the best cough suppressant ever) and made up heroin-based mixtures for severe pain relief (mostly cancer).

Knowing the ban would mean the end of this, I heard the Austin Hospital was appealing for heroin supplies to use in their cancer wards, so I donated our whole stock to them (probably illegal to do so but at least dying cancer patients could go out pain-free, having nice, probably weird dreams).

That ban on heroin started the rot, with other drugs still being banned to this day in a pointless and damaging attempt to criminalise and demonise all street drugs and drug users. As in the past, there was little or no thought or effort put into thinking about the social conditions that led many people into addiction, petty crime, poverty, sickness and death.

Later, other drugs joined the forbidden list. All cannabis preparations went - even though they are still an outstanding palliative treatment for cancer pain. The marijuana plant in all shapes and forms was banned and criminalised, as well as amphetamines of all types. The propaganda and mis-information about the evils of all these drugs was astounding. I have already referred to "Reefer Madness" which is simply laughable, but there have been a succession of learned and scientific articles, desperately trying to link marijuana with psychosis. No doubt an occasional pot smoker could develop psychotic tendencies, but so too could tobacco smokers and heavy drinkers.

With amphetamines, a central nervous system stimulant of limited value, the ban effectively gave control to bikie gangs and other citizens. They built their meth labs up in them-thar hills, abducted a few nerdy chemists (not me) and churned out methyl amphetamine ("speed") by the tonne. They also jacked up the price by a few thousand per cent. Before the ban, legal amphetamines could be bought by pharmacists for a few dollars per thousand tablets. After the ban, the prices went through the roof, particularly the designer drugs like crystal meth, ecstasy and MDA.

Cocaine was banned as well— I have never been happy about this drug. It was an excellent anaesthetic and we used it to make up very effective eye drops (cocaine and adrenaline eye drops were in every first-aid kit for treatment of painful eye injuries, particularly in industry). As a street drug, it probably did contribute to some psychosis (especially in the form of "crack") but its use seemed to be mainly confined to wealthy socialites, celebrity criminals and business people. Pot smokers and heroin users were in the lower socio-economic classes, so the full force of the law was directed at them.

There is (and always has been) a very good case to decriminalise marijuana and heroin use. The knee-jerk banning, propaganda and feigned horror about these two drugs has simply promoted corruption in police forces and the judiciary, encouraged petty crime and un-necessary sickness, misery and death. Pure heroin (and pure opiates in general) can be used for long periods of time with only minimal side-effects (probably less than just about every legally-prescribed drug).

Addicts I Have Known

As heroin took off here, we started to get many young people asking for syringes and needles. Either coincidently or in response to increased demand, disposable syringes with needles became available. At first, they were marketed for the ever-increasing diabetic population, but our street druggies soon realised they were cheap, safe and effective in minimising AIDS and hepatitis. I decided very early on to supply them in lots of five, also supplying antiseptic wipes and water for injection amps if asked. My idea was to give the young purchasers some structure to their lives. This seemed to work as many became regulars. I had no control over what they were purchasing on the street, but at least they could obtain cheap and clean equipment at regular intervals from a non-judgmental source. The official Pharmacy Board policy at the time was to condemn all illicit drug use and people like me who they considered were encouraging addiction. I never felt this was the case, and still don't, so my perfectly legal actions (though probably un-ethical to some minds) continued right up to the time I retired.

We eventually became quite busy supplying our pet addicts, and we were also one of the first pharmacies to become involved in Methadone programs. Methadone is a synthetic opiate which blocks the desire for heroin, but is more damaging than pure heroin, just as addictive and causes serious liver and kidney problems. Again, supplying cheap methadone at regular times (sometimes free) enabled some of the addicts to develop structure and routine in their lives, stay heroin-free and ease financial and health worries.

Our first two regular methadone users were quite good for a while, until the female user became erratic and revisited heroin. We also had a break-in with the stored methadone doses being stolen. I knew she had done it but said nothing (we had many break-ins over the years, all drug-related). One day, she came in shaking, pale and frantic, and asked for some emergency morphine. I slipped her a couple of tablets (which I knew I could account for by using some creative book-work). She later came back for more, but this time I said "No". This spurred her to flash a breast or two with the promise of more to come. I had heard stories about pharmacists being lured, tempted and entangled in sexual offers, with consequent blackmail, so her kind offer was declined.

Another of our female clients became a regular for a while. She was quiet, polite, charming and smart and we got on well. One day, she came in after quite a long break, and bought a syringe. She told me she had been off the stuff for a long time, but it was her birthday and she deserved a treat. A few hours later, two policemen arrived, carrying one of our paper bags. She had collapsed and died in the toilets over the road after a lethal and accidental overdose. The police stormed in, waving the bag and thinking they had cornered "Mr.Big". I simply told them what I knew (and that I had charged her an extortionate 40 cents for the syringe). They glared at me with one of the plods accusing me of complicity, while I wrote out a report and signed it. I suppose I could have been in trouble over "duty of care" concerns here, and felt dreadful that this lovely young girl had died, but I had supplied clean equipment- someone else had supplied the lethal dose.

One of our regulars was a kid with green hair who would skateboard down the middle of the busy street outside, always naked from the waist up no matter what the weather. He would zoom into the shop, buy his syringes and then skate off again. Another was a bloke who raced greyhounds and doped them up nearly as much as he doped himself. He staggered in one morning dressed in his pyjamas and whispered, "Can you help me?" He dropped his pants and I saw the pyjama cord wrapped tightly around his genitals, which had gone purple to match the color of his face. The face whitened when I brandished some tweezers and scissors, so I sighed heavily, gritted my teeth and un-knotted the cord by hand. Like Androcles when he removed a thorn from a lion's paw, I was his friend forever. Another young bloke bolted into the shop one morning, completely naked, dashed out the back and hid under a bench. He was closely followed by two paramedics who told me they had found him unconscious in the bath and slapped him around a bit to revive him.

Brendan and Neil were cousins, and came in often for their Rohypnol. They were always laughing and happy (and high), but used to disappear for months at a time. I finally asked them about their absences and they told me they had regular "holidays" in prison. They did this deliberately, getting picked up for minor possession and dealing offences. While in prison, they would eat well, be out of the cold, still get their drugs (from the warders) and Brendan, who was built like a brick shit-house, would make sure no harm came to his smaller and gentler cousin.

Glen was what some people would call a typical druggie- skinny, toothless, shifty and a smart-arse. I, of course, liked him—he co-owned a racehorse and told me when it was going to win or lose. He sometimes worked as a brickie, telling me that his bosses were all money-grubbing bastards. One night, he appeared for his methadone dose and I was surprised to see him walk out towards a Mercedes parked outside. Since he usually drove clapped out Commodores (and was always being pulled up by the police), I asked him what was going on. He grinned and said—"That lousy boss has refused to pay me and he hasn't had time to check his garage".

Ross was an ex-thug and stand - over man who had developed hepatitis C. He was now pretty sick, no longer fearsome but still dumb. He was a regular methadone patient, quite unlikeable, but constantly entertaining. He lost his driving licence but this didn't stop him stealing a car and driving to the hospital to get his weekend doses (we were strictly Monday to Saturday). This car broke down and he scalded himself badly by removing the radiator cap while it was boiling hot. Back to hospital again, this time by pushbike (also stolen) for treatment but, on the way home, he crashed over a gutter and broke his ankle. Back to the hospital again, this time by ambulance (he didn't have to steal this).

He was just starting to come good when he was shot in the shoulder in a drug deal (stolen) and pushed down some stairs. He was a constant disaster, always on the make but my main memory of him was when he broke down and cried on my shoulder after his grandfather died (in Calabria).

Another memory was him being involved in the only time I was held up at the point of a gun. A slimy little turd burst in just as we were closing, pulled a pistol out of his jacket and made me empty the contents of the drug safe. He wasn't one of "my" druggies, and I later found out that Ross was waiting outside in the getaway car (stolen). Ross later told me he didn't know I was working that night and sort of apologised by telling me the name of the bandit. I soon realised he was lying, giving me a false name to give to the police just to protect himself. I didn't really care and didn't pass on anything he told me.

As I mention addicts I've known, it will become apparent there is no stereotypical case. The young, thin, toothless and un-shaved derelict promoted by the police, the media and opportunistic politicians is a myth. Indeed it could be argued that a "typical" drug addict would be a doctor, a nurse or a pharmacist—they all have access to hard drugs, and statistics show they form a high percentage of all drug addicts.

Locum doctors, nurses and pharmacists have the worst record—they move from place to place, making detection hard, but they all eventually slip up. Alcoholism, another addiction, is also common. My father employed a locum for many years, knowing he was an alcoholic. He would hide away all the alcohol products in the shop—AB Tonic wine, Wincarnis wine, Sherry-type wine (all used as somewhat spurious "tonic" medicines) and the 95% pure alcohol all pharmacies had for making up tinctures and other extracts. This worked for a while until one of the shop assistants told my father that the locum would appear after lunch with pink lips. This was because he was getting stuck into Tincture Cardamom Co, a useful red-coloured anti-flatulence agent (with strong alcohol content).

My father had to let him go, reluctantly, because he was a good man and pharmacist, but at least he wouldn't suffer from burping and flatulence. Years later, one of my locum pharmacists, also a good worker, did the same, with one of the girls reporting that he was always blotto after his long lunches.

For some time, a gentle and polite bloke would come in, present prescriptions for his wife for pethidine or morphine, and talk to me about her pain and suffering, often crying. I always listened, sympathised and offered suggestions for alternative cancer treatments. I finally had cause to ring her doctor about a slight mistake on a script, and this is where the truth was revealed. The doctor, a psychiatrist, was horrified saying that the bloke was also a doctor and an ex-addict, and that all the scripts were forgeries. I was usually pretty good at picking forgeries (usually choosing to either ignore them or have a quiet word to the forger, telling him to go away--- of course, I was supposed to report all forgeries to the police or the Poisons Department). The psychiatrist told me I had to inform the police. I had no choice then - my wish was just to have a talk to this bloke, telling him I knew about his imaginary wife with the imaginary cancer and to congratulate him on his superb forgeries and dramatic acting.

So, the next time he bowled in, I made some pretext about waiting for the drug to be delivered. He wandered off and I rang the local police. When he came back, I sent a signal to the cops who were now parked just outside. They came in and our fabulous forger bolted out into the street and disappeared due North, chased by two red-faced, overweight cops. They didn't have a hope as this Usain Bolt of the drug world faded into the distance. Another cop in a car finally picked him up and dragged him back into the shop. All this time our latest work-experience girl was staring wide-eyed and wondering if this was a normal pharmacy. I believe this poor bloke copped a gaol sentence for all this, which is a perfect illustration of the insanity of our drug laws.

For all the trouble they gave me, I had endless patience and concern for all these people. They actually were the ones who constantly supported me in my battles. Stephen was a gentle soul, grateful for the cheap Rohypnol and my interest in him, and he leapt to my defence when another druggie was sprawled all over the counter, dribbling ice cream, demanding some serepax and being obnoxious and loud. Stephen went red, grabbed him and bundled him out the door.

I continued working after this for another 12 years, part-time and at night, until I decided the wear and tear of 50 years in Pharmacy was enough. Again, the people most upset at my departure were the local druggies.

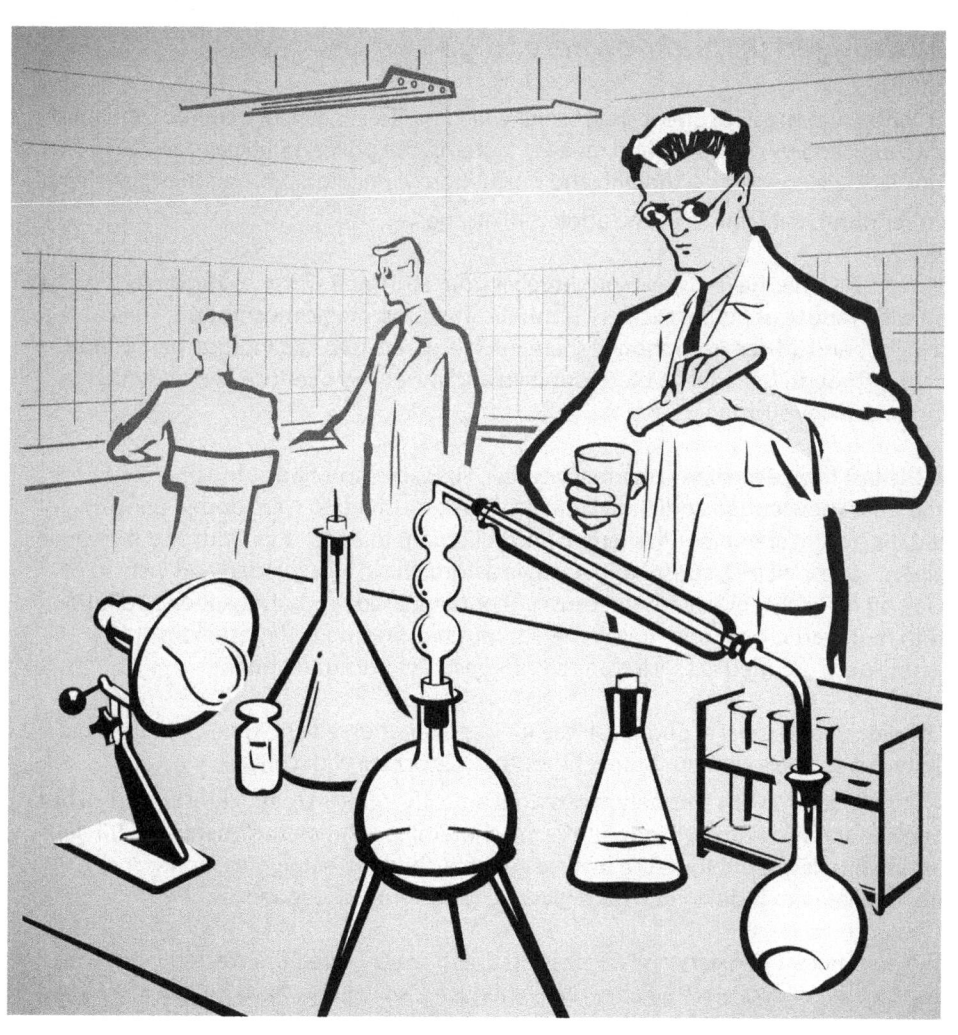

All drugged up and nowhere to go

In contrast to the illicit street drug scene which has been vilified, banned, criminalised and punished by our social and medical systems, the police, politicians and the judiciary, we now have a thriving and much more damaging promotion of "safe" legal prescription medicine, creating addicts of all ages.

Human societies have always sought relief from strife and worry by becoming hooked on wide ranges of herbal extracts, alcoholic mixtures, magic mushrooms, weird religions and advice from shonky shamans. It appears to be an integral part of human nature through the ages to block out pain and misery by over-use and addiction to just about any substance.

In the last few years of my pharmacy career, I became horrified at the unrecognised and unacknowledged addictions that proliferated. Children were doped up with sedating antihistamines (Phenergan and Vallergan) to knock them out and give their parents a rest. ADHD, autism and juvenile asthma have all exploded and instead of looking for likely environmental causes (contaminated food, atmospheric pollution with high particle content, heavy metals, routine spraying with pesticides and herbicides), our medical system, as always, resorts to drug treatment.

The easiest and most economical way for our over-stressed and time-poor medical system is to mess with our brain-chemistry. This occurs with children who are routinely doped with amphetamines from an early age to treat ADHD and other behavioural syndromes. In adults, the amphetamines and methylphenidate (Ritalin) act as stimulants, but have the reverse effect in children, helping to sedate and tranquillise with little or no regard given to long-term consequences.

The epidemics of anxiety and depression that have engulfed the Western world are also treated with drugs that alter brain chemistry, so we now have people of all ages being experimented on. In the bad old days (which weren't all that bad really), "mental illness" and "nervous breakdowns" were treated with drugs that truly zombified the patients, and induced horrific dyskinesias and ataxias, and the unfortunate sufferers were isolated in horrific institutions (safely locked away from our "healthy" society). The newer generation of drugs are much safer, but they still play havoc with serotonin, dopamine and nor-adrenalin. These all take part in a continual, finely balanced dance in the brain, constantly being produced, destroyed and removed in micro fractions of a second. Using drugs to alter this balance is hopelessly clumsy and eventually damaging.

All anatomical and physiological systems are incredibly complex and fine-tuned. The immune system, the nerve-muscle synapses mediated by acetyl choline and cholinesterase, the liver-enzyme system and the already mentioned brain chemistry system have developed over millennia, so drug treatment on these systems is hopelessly inadequate. Ideally, there should always be a holistic approach — that is, treatment by doctors of the WHOLE organism, not just the particular system that has broken down (which explains the dominance and proliferation of medical specialists who know everything about their tiny field of expertise, and nothing about the complete, holistic organism).

Now we come to the worst cases of all – the treatment of the elderly. The inmates of nursing homes are truly drugged up to their eyeballs and being turned into addicts by constant dosing with benzodiazepines—Valium, Serepax, Xanax during the day and Temazepam and Nitrazepam at night. The whole economic-based model is based on modern families having neither the time, money or concern to look after their elders. It is truly shameful that our modern, wealthy society takes this option when other so-called more primitive and deprived societies care for their elders respectfully and with dignity.

So, this is the pattern of modern-day addictions. They are all caused (and even promoted) by self-interest and the profit motive, whereby vast quantities of drugs are demanded by our worried, anxious, depressed and frightened people who demand to stay healthy and to live for ever. Naturally, the drugs are duly supplied, with no thought or energy being given to address the social and environmental disintegration that is causing all the problems.

Grannies, Drugs and Money

Of all new drugs released, 25% have serious safety issues. Relating to toxicology, most poisonings admitted to hospitals are from prescription drugs.

Granny drug pushers

Sedatives, hypnotics and pain-killers top the list with there being a sharp rise in the use and abuse of oxycodone, an opiate. I have just read that dear old grannies are selling their Endone, Oxy-contin, Oxy-norm and MS-Contin on the street to teenage drug fiends in order to bankroll their poker machine addictions.

Overdosing and poisoning from street drugs – heroin, the amphetamines, marijuana —is smaller and almost entirely due to uncertain purity and strength (a problem solved immediately by de-criminalising and then regulating). The soaring crime rates would also disappear and the police would have to concentrate on gambling for their bribes and corruption.

Alarming bath poisonings

The alarming news is the increase in poisoning from 'psychoactive bath salts'. I think this was originally a clever and sneaky way to distribute amphetamines in bath salts, which were then sold openly. I presume the poisoning has come from those who drink their own bath water.

CONTRACEPTION

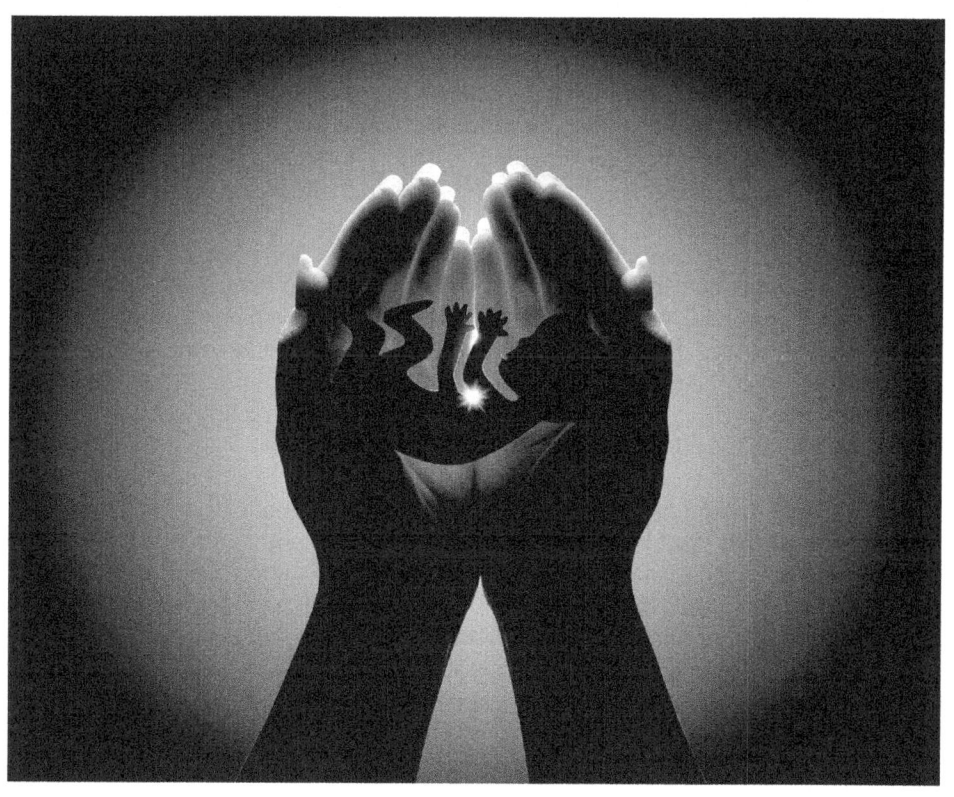

To Be Or Not To Be - That is the QES-tion?

The story of abortion law reform in Australia is a long and shameful one. My grandfather and father (and later me) always kept substantial stocks of QES tablets. This seemed strange to me at first since they were a schedule 4 drug – that is, they required a doctor to write a prescription before they could be supplied. In my fifty year career (and also in my father's time) I never saw one doctor's prescription for this item and the reason for the stocks of QES tablets in most pharmacies soon became clear.

They were a crafty combination of Quinine, Ergot and Strychnine designed to induce uterine contractions. Quinine and strychnine had been used for years in small doses as tonics (they had a bitter taste so they must have been good). Quinine was also a treatment for malaria, muscle cramps, fevers in general and even a pessary - based spermicide contraceptive.

Like all the drugs developed from botanical sources over many years, quinine and the other alkaloids derived from cinchona bark were extremely useful drugs. Ergot, developed from a fungus growing on rye grass, was used in obstetrics to promote contractions and to treat post-partum haemorrhage. It was also extremely useful and potent and, as a liquid extract, was administered by pharmacists - not doctors - to induce abortion.

The ergot alkaloids became very effective treatments for migraine and were made into one of the greatest compounds of all time - LSD or lysergic acid di-ethylamide. Strychnine was derived from the Nux Vomica plant and was mainly used as a rat poison and a convenient plot device for Agatha Christie stories (a mysterious white crystalline powder was always discovered by Miss Marple in the shed in the last few pages of the book—the wife or the mistress was always the murderer).

So, in my grandfather's time, QES pills were formulated and made up in the pharmacy, using quaint old pill machines. The doses of the quinine, ergot and strychnine were carefully worked out, the idea being there was sufficient to abort the foetus (sorry all you right-to-lifers) by inducing uterine contractions without harming the woman. As a corollary to furtive men sneaking in and asking for the shameful French letters etc., this industry relied on furtive women having long and earnest talks with the pharmacist before the pills would be put into an un-labelled bottle, directions given (one pill three times daily for four days) and money changing hands (not a fortune to be made here - I can remember my father charging three bob the lot).

When I started in 1958 as an apprentice to my father, we no longer used the pill machine. The QES tablets could be purchased through wholesale drug companies in lots of 100 and doled out as before (still cheap). I believe they were quite effective with only the odd failure. Management afterwards relied on common sense, with any women suffering persistent or copious bleeding advised to seek immediate medical help. I think most pharmacists balanced out the risks and the illegality of these practices pretty well. It was a dismal scene with desperate, pregnant women fighting against poverty, ignorance, religious intolerance and corruption (police were notoriously involved in protecting the 'back-yard abortionists' who had a terrible record of botched procedures, infections, high cost and strange uses of knitting needles).

There were no hospitals and very few doctors who would offer any help, so the women were forced to drink copious amounts of castor oil while sitting in a scalding hot bath or falling down some stairs. I believe pharmacists were uncomfortable with this cruel system, but when faced with desperately poor and down-trodden pregnant women, felt obliged to help, and good old QES was cheap, safe and relatively effective.

There were never any pharmacists actively advertising themselves as "your friendly local abortionist", but the QES story was obviously spread by word of mouth, and to me, it was the best and perhaps the only, option for women who couldn't face up to un-wanted pregnancy. One more strange thing about QES was the complete lack of any written information about it. In this day of rampant over-information about everything - face-booking, twittering, tweeting, and You-Tubing us all into glassy-eyed trivialised zombies, there were no mentions of QES in any of the many medical or drug text books. The information about composition, dosage, usage and side-effects (now mandatory for all drugs) simply didn't exist. It was truly a 'peoples' drug, handed down by osmosis through the ages, courtesy of your friendly local abortionist—sorry – pharmacist.

Other ancient abortofacients and emmenogogues (menstruation-inducing) included pennyroyal, slippery elm powder, wormwood and other anthelmintics and many other botanical derivatives, none of which were as effective as QES and often being quite toxic to the women.

My next contribution will move on to the turbulent 1960's when a few brave people fought against venality, greed, corruption and stupidity to achieve abortion law reform.

You Wouldn't Conceive of It

The long, tawdry and depressing tale of Australia's (and particularly Victoria's) continual ignoring of women's security and health didn't change much until the 1960's. For years, police had been involved in kick-backs, bribes, protection rackets and covering up the so-called victimless crimes. These were illegal betting, (SP bookies down every lane in the suburbs), prostitution and brothels (next door to the SP bookies), illegal gambling in pubs and clubs, and illegal drinking and sly-grog shops. These all flourished in a State that pretended they weren't there – in our dull and conformist suburban wastelands, no-one ever mentioned drinking, smoking, gambling or the sex trade, including abortion. It was a climate of fear, repression and silence.

The back-yard abortionists were thriving (even if their customers often didn't), with the police protecting them and getting well paid for their trouble. This changed when a few brave and progressive individuals challenged the system. A nurse, Peggy Berman, and a retired cop, Jack Herbert, accused some high-ranking police of corruption. This followed on from Doctor Bertram Wainer and his wife Jo, openly encouraging women to come to them for their still illegal terminations. The full weight of the legal, political and religious systems descended upon them, but with the evidence of Berman and Jack "The Bagman" Herbert (who delivered cash from the back-yarders to the police), a Royal Commission was finally instigated.

They found that many police, including three police inspectors, had for years been raking off thousands of pounds in bribes. I knew one of the inspectors – Jack Matthews – who was a local Fairfield boy who had worked his way to the top. I felt some pity but knew he was part of wide-spread corruption causing extreme suffering and misery. He was just taking advantage of the mess created by politics, religion and the law. He and two others were jailed for 5 years or so, but the important thing was the change in public attitudes to abortion.

Bert and Jo Wainer continued, still under duress and threats (contracts were taken out on their lives at one stage) and, with a favourable court ruling, abortions could at last be legally and safely performed. Bert Wainer died from a heart attack soon after and Jo Wainer continued his work, establishing the Melbourne Fertility Clinic where nowadays you can still see the Right-to-Lifers waving placards, frothing at the mouth, shouting at and harassing women who enter the building.

If nothing else, the abortion issue illustrated the futility of the State enforcing prohibition policies for these victimless "crimes" – they are human desires and sometimes failings, but it is up to a healthy society to deal with them, not politicians, police or bible-bangers. At a later date I will describe how the State is still creating misery and despair in its "war on drugs".

From the 1960's onwards, abortion became more low key. In pharmacy, the main change was for the QES tablets to slowly disappear, to be replaced by an innovative and clever use of the contraceptive pill. Someone, somewhere, somehow (I think these things sometimes arise via the collective unconscious) discovered that a larger dose would act to induce abortion. Instead of taking one tablet per day, the dose was upped to two tablets every 12 hours. A brand called 'Nordiol' was the favourite. Again, few doctors would ever order "the pill" in such a fashion but, as with QES, most pharmacists would have stocks of 'Nordiol' on hand, ready to sneak out 4 tablets (from a pack of 21), when required. It had few side effects used like this, was very effective and again, very cheap.

Eventually this underground method was legitimised and formalised by the creation of the "morning after pill". This formulation simply upped the dosage into one pill, placed two tablets in a fancy packet, with copious warnings, instructions and counselling, and was distributed and marketed by your friendly foreign drug cartel with a 50-fold increase in price.

This has been a major advance in safe, convenient oral inducement of abortion with perhaps the only unfortunate side-effect being many young girls becoming repeat-offenders. That is, go to a rave, get drunk or high, have sex and then rush into the nearest pharmacy the day after for an instant fix. I could be accused of generalising here.

The next major development should be the release of RU486 (mifepristone) as a single dose and safe treatment, though this may have to wait until religious-based negativity diminishes. Pharmacists (including my father and me) were visited by increasing numbers of women seeking contraception or abortion, because the local priests were monstering the local Catholic pharmacists. They were threatened with hell-fire and eternal damnation if they ever dared to help women in these matters. I presume the women were also threatened in this way, but being pragmatic about their (and their families') welfare, they opted for assistance from sympathetic pharmacists.

I will end this with a note of warning: Beware the concept of "Personhood". This is a deluded and cruel movement being fostered in the deep South of America by Republicans, Tea-Party fanatics and the fundamentalist religious right. Many of these Southern states have already legislated that any woman seeking an abortion MUST have a trans-vaginal ultrasound beforehand. I presume this is so they can view the embryo, think "What a beautiful looking person they are", realise the error of their ways, cancel the abortion and run screaming "Halleluiah, the Lord be praised!" to join the nearest church. No room to measure the psychological and emotional harm done to the women, already worried and perhaps confused about the moral implications.

I have no doubt that "Personhood" will at some time be foisted upon the women of Australia.

Not in My Backyard

My grandfather and father were both pharmacists, with my grandfather working from 1900 to 1945, my father from 1935 to 1962 and me from 1961 to 2010, so we have covered a century or more. My grandfather was very versatile, travelling around country towns as a locum pharmacist and as an occasional emergency dentist. During his and my father's time, women were often victims of cruel, patriarchal and legalistic policies of oppression regarding birth control and abortion.

During those early times of war, the Great Depression and poverty, women suffered a great deal, with minimal birth control available. There were condoms for the men (if they could be bothered) and some rather weird and wonderful pessary-like contraptions for women. One of these was a strange combination of fibres forming a sponge which featured in an hilarious Seinfeld episode where Elaine discovered a whole carton of them at an ancient pharmacy run by an equally ancient pharmacist. She bought the lot (for a lifetime's supply) and proceeded to ration them out carefully by pre-determining whether her latest partner was "sponge-worthy" or not.

Spermicide gels and creams emerged later and were applied to pessaries or diaphragms. However, they were messy and inconvenient as well as being "cides" which means they killed living cells with unknown consequences to other living tissue.
So, in these hard times, women had large families and lived in a constant state of insecurity and poverty. Some of these contraceptives had names like "Ortho-Gynol" jelly and cream - sounds like it wouldn't be out of place at a fancy restaurant - "Delfen" cream and foam, "Preceptin" gel and "Rendells Pessaries". Women who could afford it were measured up and fitted with diaphragms by their friendly GPs (gently and with warm hands we hope). They then carried them around in dinky little purses, ever-ready for their next encounter.

When I started in pharmacy, I was bewildered by all the names for condoms. The word "condom" was seldom used; instead, men would sidle in, head for the nearest male attendant and mumble out of the corner of their mouths. They'd ask for a pack of French letters or Sheaths or Checkers or Super Checkers (for preventing the birth of super heroes?) or Wet-Chex or Check-mate (where you resign and concede defeat?) or Durex - they had this name before the sticky-tape people pinched it, with many embarrassing consequences later on - or prophylactics or rubbers or simply " frangas".

These purchases were always conducted in silence; no eye contact and a large amount of stuttering and red faces for it was a shameful secret that such things existed. They were always stored in draws below the counter, so to see today's gaudy displays in modern pharmacies – bright colours, different shapes and sizes, weird appendages, glow-in-the-dark, scented, lubricated, singing, talking, dancing and exploding (for the true thrill-seeker) - is truly an amazing turnaround.

In the 1960's, the next development in contraception was "the pill" (how quickly this became the accepted and iconic terminology).

Pill - Oh Talk

Before we lurch into the 1960's, free love, psychodelia and "the Pill", mention must be made of the brilliant contribution made to contraceptive practices by "Vatican Roulette". The Catholic church had been quietly promoting this for years and now, with the advent of oral contraceptives, they really pushed it hard, fearing that wild debauchery would descend upon good Catholic women if they took "the Pill".

This fabulously unsuccessful method involved taking accurate body temperatures, which varied according to the time of ovulation each month. The theory was that there were optimal times to either become pregnant or optimal times to avoid pregnancy. All over the world there were huge numbers of Catholic women either saying "Bugger- I'm pregnant" or "Bugger- I'm not pregnant". Still, Vatican Roulette was a cheap method with minimal side-effects (the occasional un-wanted child or two) and is still being promoted.

The combined oestrogen/progesterone pill was indeed a revolution but one that again ignored or down-played side-effects on women. It ticked all the boxes (how I hate that term) regarding convenience (for men), cost and safety (up to a point) but, as with HRT, it soon emerged that risk of stroke and heart problems could occur.

Over the years, different combinations of hormones were tried (and in ever decreasing doses) which eased some of the risks, but the fact remained that once again a natural hormonal cycle in women was being artificially altered. It sometimes worked well in regulating erratic or painful cycles in a small percentage of women, which I have no real problem with. However, the mass marketing of "the Pill" was based more on socio-economic grounds than medical ones.

More women were joining the work force each year and needed to be not pregnant every two years or so, and since men were not going to be responsible, have vasectomies or be experimented on with hormone treatment, women were conned, coerced and brainwashed into tinkering with their natural reproductive systems.

The listed side-effects of any drug can be frightening and overwhelming—these are tabulated on a statistical basis, listing common, frequent and rare effects - and I believe each drug-taking person should be aware of these. However, we must also realise everyone is an individual with individual and unique liver and kidney systems (these are the organs directly involved in drug metabolism, break-down and excretion). These systems are genetically driven and then modified throughout a person's life by their particular environment. For example, liver enzyme systems can be upset by herbicides, pesticides, heavy metals, alcohol abuse and many other factors.

I suppose the message I am trying to convey is to respect your own natural systems and try not to interfere with them by using any drugs at all. Of course, moderation is always the key – I know some drugs are useful (even essential) at times. I have the greatest admiration for the skills of surgeons, nurses, shamans, witch-doctors, yogis, gurus (some of them – the ones who don't drive around in gold-plated Mercedes or have harems) and even the odd doctor who is not hell-bent on drug-peddling.

CANCER

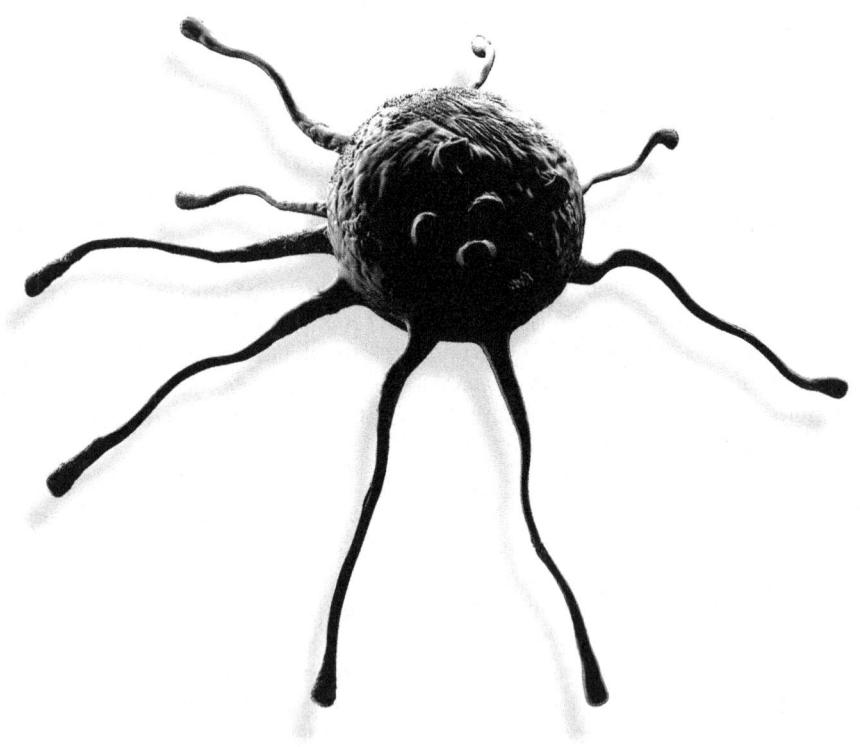

Why we need a new attitude to cancer

Cancer is a natural function

The treatment and attitude toward cancer in our society is a sad story.

I realise it is completely understandable that doctors and families of cancer patients will promote aggressive drug treatment and radiotherapy.

Our attitude may change, however, if cancer were to be viewed not as a disease, but as a natural function of all cell-based life.

Cells have finite life spans

All cells have finite life spans.

They grow, live and die to a strict time-line and have a "killer" gene which switches them off at the right time.

Cancer cells, where the killer gene malfunctions, arise in every organism and are usually destroyed by the immune system.

Environmental degradation compromising our immune systems

But, largely due to our mismanagement, the environment is rapidly degrading.

This degradation amplifies the naturally occurring carcinogens such as viruses, atmospheric particles, radiation, tobacco, asbestos, a wide range of chemicals and probably many unknown factors. What then happens is that our immune systems fail and cancers arise.

Cancer is a natural consequence of aging and aging cells are more likely to malfunction. Of course, cancer can strike at any age which only illustrates the complexity and randomness of this life function.

I repeat: cancer is **NOT** a disease.

Yet we spend a fortune treating it like it is.

Disturbing information about new cancer drugs

Some recent information about the cost of new drugs to treat cancer is disturbing.

A drug used to treat leukaemia in the elderly has been approved at a cost of $5000 per month for each patient, because it has been shown to increase the median survival rate by 7 months compared to 5 months using placebo.

A drug used to treat metastatic colon cancer increased the median survival rate by 1.4 months, but cost $11,000 per month. This was actually greeted by a few howls of outrage and it was replaced by a drug only costing $6000 per month.

Our fear of death drives this drug insanity

While our society has such a fear of death and is driven by an insane desire to stay healthy forever, these absurdities will continue.

Even Australia's one-time richest man, the late Kerry Packer, supplying himself with his very own MICA ambulance and seemingly having an inexhaustible supply of helicopter pilots willing to donate an organ or two, couldn't bribe the Grim Reaper to look the other way.

Over-diagnosis another sorry cancer story

Another recent report concerns the dangers of over-diagnosis.

With constant screening for breast cancer, cervical cancer, prostate cancer, bowel cancer and other cancers of the month, more cancers are being detected.

On the surface, this is a good thing, the orthodoxy being early detection means early treatment and saved lives. Look beyond the "early-detection saves lives" orthodoxy, however, and you will discover that many of these cancers will not kill you in the first place.

So many, in fact, that oncologists call them "incidental-omas".

It has been estimated that for every woman who doesn't die of breast cancer because of screening, three are over-diagnosed and subsequently over-treated with the usual distressing side-effects of chemotherapy.

Mini health report: The cancers that won't kill you

Medical over – diagnosis

Another recent report concerns the dangers of over-diagnosis. With constant screening for breast cancer, cervical cancer, prostate cancer, bowel cancer and other "cancers of the month", more cancers are being detected.

On the surface, this is a good thing, the orthodoxy being early detection means early treatment and saved lives. However, there are now many cancers being detected that will not kill you, so many in fact, that oncologists call them "incidental-omas".

It has been estimated that for every woman who doesn't die of breast cancer because of screening, three are over-diagnosed and subsequently over-treated (with the usual distressing side-effects of chemotherapy).

Our "War on Drugs" has deadly ramifications

A deadly combination of the Western world's "war on drugs", and its monopoly on the opiate pain-killing drugs, has meant that 90% of the world's morphine is used in affluent countries while pain goes un-treated in Asian, African and South American countries. It is almost impossible to obtain morphine in India.

Why Cannabis should be used in cancer treatments

Recent articles promote the idea of marijuana being used as a cancer treatment.

This is a valid idea as the cannabinoids (the active ingredients of cannabis) have anti-inflammatory and anti-cancer effects — they induce death of cancer cells. There will be no investigation into this from the big pharmaceutical companies, since there will be no money in it for them.

Cannabis is cheap, grows like a weed and probably can't be patented. Trials on animals and then people, are very expensive, so Bigpharma devotes all its time to developing "Mabs" and "Nibs" to treat cancer. These cost a fortune and are protected by 10 year patents, so that all the shareholders are rejoicing as the money rolls in.

They aren't all that successful either— you often read heart-rending stories of melanoma sufferers who can't afford the huge amounts of money required, so a public fund is set up (by the media, but they don't contribute). They may extend a life by 3 to 6 months – all with horrendous side-effects – but it is a great story for the media and the publicity is good for Bigpharma.

Doctors and cancer specialists are financed by Bigpharma to attend seminars on their latest "life-saving" drug, usually in Vanuatu, Hawaii or the Swiss alps. The "life-saving" drug is then heavily promoted (only favourable reviews, of course, from all those doctors when they return from their vacation—sorry — seminar).

Unfavourable reviews are never mentioned

I believe Cannabis and its extracts would have a better effect on cancer than all the overpriced drugs from Bigpharma, particularly when you take the placebo effect into consideration.

Smoking pot is not so good (lung cancer is a possibility), but the old cannabis extracts and tinctures could be marketed, and made into recipes. I see that in Colorado they now have hash cookies, hash chocolate and hash marmalade.

At least, even if this doesn't work all the time, people will be a lot happier as they nibble on a hash chocolate.

HEALTH

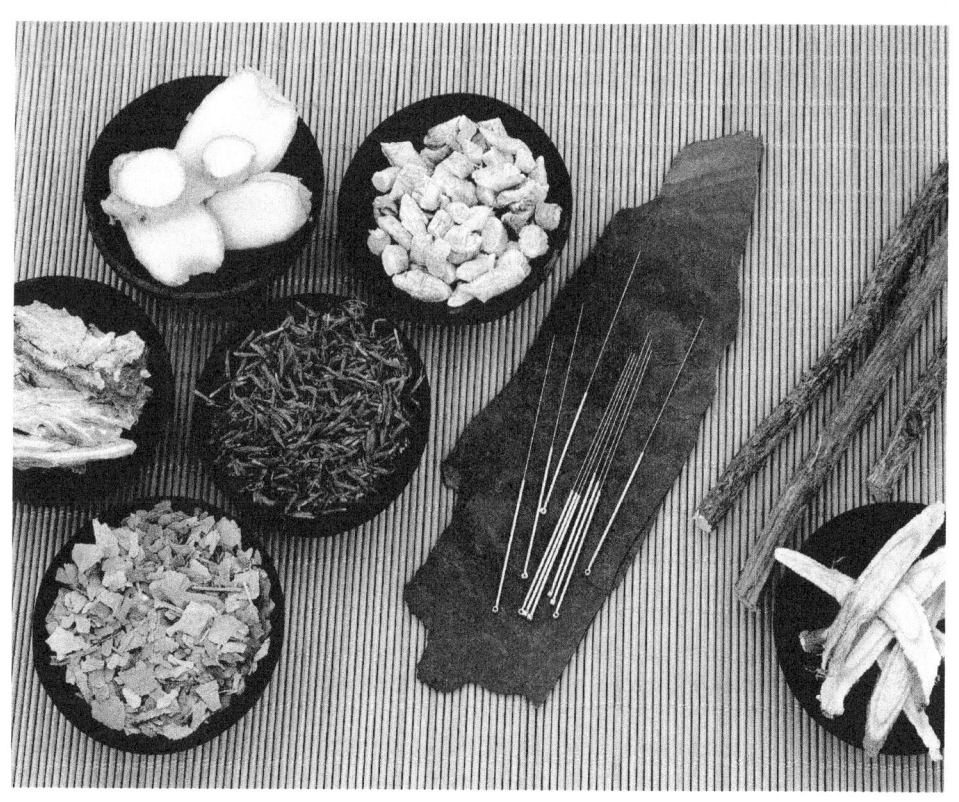

Why our food is making us sick

A big reason many of us are so sick is the purity of our food.

That is, most foods we eat these days are too pure.

A diet of sea salt or rock salt has many trace elements, but purified salt (pure Sodium Chloride) may contribute to high blood pressure and kidney failure.

Fats and sugars are also over-purified. High sucrose, glucose or fructose in pure form could explain the obesity and diabetic epidemic. Raw brown cane sugar and fructose from fruits and vegetables (coupled with trace elements, fibre, tannin and vitamins), would be much safer than all the junk-food that people now eat.

Children are especially vulnerable and on a pathway to obesity and ill health. Purified fructose and corn syrup – with the added attraction of being genetically modified — now abound in Coca-Cola, cereals and canned foods, all heavily advertised and directed towards children. Diet coke and diet Pepsi, with aspartame as the un-natural sweetener, have now been linked to weight gain because they sharpen our appetite and make us eat more because of the psychological catch of the word "diet" in the brand names.

Aspartame, by the way, was a by-product of an anti-cancer drug a few years ago, and now it is being linked to cancer itself.

Saturated fat and cholesterol have been panned by doctors ever since the 1950s. Now it seems that these aren't the villains. To supply a person's daily calorie count, saturated fat is the best option, from animal or vegetable sources. Butter, cheese and other dairy products are also good. We have been scared into using margarine, which dieticians hate because it has no nutritional value and tastes like sludge, and told to replace saturated fat with carbohydrates, and this is why diabetes is raging.

Aborigines in Australia never suffered from diabetes until they were paid with refined flour, sugar, tobacco and grog and now they have one of the highest rates of diabetes in the world.

We now use unsaturated fats, all refined and purified instead of unrefined fat from many sources. We have been brainwashed into only using extra-virgin olive oil – virgin olive oil, or just plain olive oil, doesn't seem to exist.

In other words, we should exist as our ancestors did and eat a wide range of unrefined food from animals and vegetables with the proviso that too much is bad for you, and that too much of any particular food could also be bad for you.

Human health sniffles towards Bethlehem

As human health worsens in all directions, our answer is to spend billions of dollars on cures for cancer, cardiovascular disease, diabetes, autism and ADHD, the last two of which are now epidemics in the young.

Modern drug treatment is a (very) expensive sham. Our aim should be prevention of illness by regulating environment — removal of pesticides, herbicides, heavy metals, coal dust, and other air particles – and to stop our rat-race style of existence which, under threat from human population growth, has made us demented and unhinged.

So-called mental illness is increasing rapidly among all age groups. I would prefer mental "illness" to be called a human failing of spirit, mind and soul. This can only be corrected by improving the conditions under which we live. Spending money on drugs is futile and only lines the pockets of Big Pharma and leaves medical orthodoxy trailing behind, fearful of litigation from Big Pharma's team of lawyers.

We are now even thinking of ovarian transplants to increase fertility for an already over-populated world. This is madness, as is IVF which costs thousands of dollars for each one month treatment.

One of the big worries at present is the risk of contagion. At one end of the scale, crèches, pre-schools and kindergartens have flourished (or at least the people running them have). Strange, contagious diseases now spread very rapidly – slapped cheek syndrome, hand, foot and mouth disease (foot and mouth only occur in sheep and cattle), Molluscum Contagiosum and other bacterial and viral ailments. These then spread to parents and (particularly) grandparents.

Molluscum Contagiosum (MCV) has now spread everywhere in the contagion factories (crèches, schools, etc.). It will always clear up in one or two weeks, but worried parents want results right now. A cream, Imimiquod which was developed for skin cancers, is now used extensively for MCV. It costs $20 and has the same effect as covering the lesions with sticky tape. Hand, foot and mouth, which was always a mild viral infection, has now morphed into something more serious, affecting livers and kidneys.

On the other end of the scale is the proliferation of nursing homes. Here, we see depression, psychosis, Alzheimer's disease (now expected to affect 33% of all American citizens) and bi-polar disorder.

As previously stated, we have a huge failing of spirit, mind and soul, which is completely environmental. Every nursing home patient is on laxatives due to side-effects of all the drugs they are on, and outbreaks of scabies occur every few months or so. They are given opioids during the day and sedated at night.

This is the society we have become — children and old people have been institutionalised and we have created infection factories. Michael Leunig in The Age a few years ago, drew a cartoon that showed kids in a detention centre. He was howled down and criticised by (mostly) working mothers. Leunig and I aren't working mothers, but we still despair.

Why the diet industry is a big fat rip-off

We are genetically programmed to be of certain shape.

Big, small, large bones, small bones, fat, chunky, lumpy, obese, skinny, slender or skeletal and from birth it depends on how much junk food and sugary drinks it takes to get an individual fat.

The fattest people are now in America, followed closely by Australia (as always), where crap foods and drinks are now linked with a complete lack of exercise, particularly in young people.

If authorities wish to stop the spread of diabetes and heart problems, they should curtail advertising from BigPharma and Big Junkfood, promote clean, uncontaminated food and water, get bums off seats by banning mobile phones and computers until the age of 30, and make children walk, horse-ride or bike-ride to and from school.

I don't think this is going too far and it won't happen anyway.

So, in the opinion of health authorities we now have miracle diets and miracle appetite suppressants.

None of these diets and appetite suppressants work.

You may lose weight at the start, but quickly resume your own body shape. What's worse, the appetite suppressants are all based on "speed", which makes you feel good as your weight drops and then rises again, possibly with associated brain damage.

Weight-loss gurus drop dead too

One of the first celebrity weight reduction gurus was Nathan Pritikin (in America of course), who designed a diet of nuts, legumes, organic fruit and cereals and other healthy stuff. He sold millions of books, all with good-looking Hollywood stars on the cover. Amazingly, these books still sold even after he jogged down a Chicago street and dropped dead at the age of 60. He may have reverted to junk food and not told anyone.

The first diet tablets

The first diet tablets to appear were Ephedrine, closely followed by Dexamphetamine and Methyl Amphetamine. These were cheap and plentiful, did a reasonable job and dieting people were always happy (but a bit crazed).

Women were the main users — as they still are today – but men stayed fat because they didn't care and no-one looked at them anyway.

Hells Angels muscle in

When our sensible health authorities (there's that bloody word again) banned the sale of amphetamines, the only way to procure some was to know a friendly Hells Angel. The price went up, purity went down but very few complained and the ones who did lost a few knee caps.

New amphetamine-based drugs now appear courtesy of BigPharma, ridiculously expensive and loaded with side-effects. Drugs such as Adifax (schizophrenia, cardiovascular effects, porphyria), Ponderax (as above, plus disturbances in heart rhythm butthey eventually banned this one), Ritalin (now being fed to children), Duromine (these now cost over $100 for one month's supply), Anorex, Tenuate and others, all at prices that could rival the Hells Angel industry and doing as much harm.

BigPharma is now pushing, with the help of the medical profession, Orlistat ("Xenical") and Sibutramine ("Reductil").
Xenical can induce vomiting and diarrhoea (a good way to lose weight), and if taken with fatty foods, can induce explosive vomiting and diarrhoea (an even better way).

Reductil is now implicated in Serotonin Syndrome, which is a serious and sometimes fatal disruption of brain chemicals. This is a real problem, especially since most people seem to be on anti-depressants (because they are over-weight). This results in an increase in the amount of serotonin in your system and nobody knows why this works for depressed people, nor the imbalances it produces.

Biggest fat rip-offs of all

The biggest rip-offs are the exotic Amazonian and Asian fat-blasters and de-tox agents, full of antioxidants, vitamins and cholesterol-lowers, sold over the counter by your friendly discount pharmacies. We have fat-blaster diuretics, fat magnets, fat busters and de-tox for liver and kidneys.

None of them work, and the manufacturers operate on the theory that the more you pay, the better it will be — well at least for them, not the customer.

The biggest rort in recent times was on American TV, where Dr Mehmet Oz promoted Raspberry Ketone,"the fat buster in a bottle."

Ketones are in many plants, minding their own business and doing a good job for their plant. They have since found that the Raspberry Ketone is extracted from rhubarb, peaches, grapes, pine trees and can be synthesized – which is where most of it comes from.

In summary, don't believe anything on TV, and treat with scepticism all diets, pronouncements from doctors and anything from BigPharma.

You can watch the Youtube video for this article at: *https://www.youtube.com/watch?v=srY8Wib-KvU*

Save on health products and suck on a tree instead

Health-related advertising by sports stars, all with an unquenchable thirst for more money and an unquenchable lack of knowledge about the products, is at a peak.

This is what washed-up cricketers, swimmers and footballers advertise on TV, radio and in newspapers:

Krill everything

Super krill oil, red krill oil, osteo krill oil, wild krill oil, deep sea krill oil, eco-krill oil (not for 'ecology' but for 'economics' as krill are harvested and sold to gullible people).

Anything with oil

Fish oil, wild fish oil — they're shitty because they got caught — calamari oil, red calamari oil, calamari 'brain-sharp' oil (I need some).

In fact, whatever you do, don't secrete oil if you're a life-form or you'll end up on a pharmacy shelf.

Vitamins for humans, grumps and Martians

Vitamins for kids, teens, men, women, Martians and grumpy old curmudgeons. They claim to improve vision (not television – but enough to see through all this rubbish), taste (but not in these ads), smell (you can smell the ads coming), touch (you get touched every time you fork out), hearing and telepathy.
Tablets for mood swings (up or down), relaxation and sleep, executive stress, executive sleep and executives getting fired (because of over-stress and under-sleep).
Advertising of kids' vitamins at rock bottom

These ads also bang on about Vita-Gummies (Calcium and Vitamin D for osteoporosis — go out into the sun, it's cheaper), Vita-Gummies with vitamins and veggies (it must be an enormous tablet to fit the cauliflour and pumpkin in), Vita-Gummies Immune Booster (hopefully, immunity against these ridiculous ads) and Vita-Gummies Something For Fussy Eaters (they don't like Big Macs or KFC).

Other useless health-product exotica

Gingko biloba which helps you to focus and remember how much money you waste on all this junk.

Melatonin, a naturally occurring "sleep" hormone, which for some reason is banned in Australia — maybe because too much sleep may force people to act rationally.
Co-enzyme Q10 at really inflated prices. This is a naturally occurring substance that is knocked out because of the doctors pushing statins onto everyone.

Fat blasters

And then they blather on about Fat Blasters

Fat Blaster diuretics (flush it down the toilet where all this stuff belongs).
Fat Magnets (I'm unsure if this is to reduce weight or gain weight but it doesn't matter because they don't work).
Fat Blaster Coconut Detox (ever seem a fat coconut?)
Fat Blaster chewing gum to reduce hunger pangs and to stop "snacking". (It belts you over the head if you go near the fridge after midnight.)

Suck on a tree

You can also pay a fortune for chlorophyll mixture and tablets, but why not suck a tree?

Complaints

The Therapeutic Goods Administration has had many complaints about false advertising directed against some of the larger pharmacies, but as is the case with the Environmental Protection Agency, the Broadcasting Control Board and other toothless tigers, no action is ever taken.

Economics is the winner here — everyone must spend no matter what the personal and environmental cost.

Meanwhile, all these worthless substances gush into our degraded oceans and poison whatever's left in them.

A holistic health system is the way forward

The more Big Pharma's drug researchers concentrate on changing every natural system in the human body, the more convinced I become of holistic medicine's many benefits.

Ultimately, drug companies prey on our fear of growing old and tell us that, with a little help from them, we can stay healthy forever.

They have tampered with brain chemistry, gut chemistry, every endocrine organ in the body, blood-pressure, cholesterol, insulin resistance and heart and lung function. This is mostly to no avail, however, as not one system can be targeted on its own. Every cell in the body is affected, and this is why side-effects are so rampant. Each drug on the market — which, by the way, is barely ahead of placebo — has side-effects ranging from not so good to absolutely catastrophic. The doctors, fearful of litigation or being de-registered by an incredibly conservative AMA, will change the brand or try something else rather than take their patients off a problematic medication.

Holistic healers are around, though, and they concentrate on exercise, sun exposure and healthy diets. They take steps to remove or minimise contaminants in food and in the air and treat the entire body, rather than bombarding individual organs with Big Pharma's poisons.

Another threat to everyone's health is the spread of "agronomics"– mostly driven by Monsanto in America and Bayer in Germany.

Monsanto is producing crops (maize, corn, soy, canola) which are genetically modified so that they are Round-up resistant. Litre upon litre of Round-up (made by Monsanto, of course) is then sprayed on rather appealing weeds.

Once all the farmers are hooked, and instead of saving some seed for next year's crop, they now have to buy GMO seed (from Monsanto, of course). Monsanto and the American Grocery Association are now suing several US states that have tried to make it compulsory for GMO labelling to occur.

Crops drenched in Round-up (Glyphosate plus dispersants and solvents) might account for the vast increase in neurological disorders, particularly in children (autism, ADHD), and many adult ailments.

The tame Monsanto scientists (similar to the scientists from the tobacco and alcohol industry) perpetuate the hoax that animals are unaffected by all this chemical bombardment. But this is untrue.

When plants grow, they rely on the Shimono process, and this is what Round-up targets in weeds. The Shimono process doesn't exist in animals, but, and it's a very big but, gut bacteria in animals is wiped out when they eat Round-up soaked plants.

Gut bacteria in humans are almost all beneficial, essential for health and, once again, should not be tampered with. Herbicides and pesticides change them markedly, as do antibiotics, treatments for diarrhoea and constipation, and now some of the u/bute treatments for excess acid secretion.

Similar to the alterations in brain chemistry caused by drugs used to treat depression, anxiety, psychosis, doctors don't seem to know why or how these drugs work. And so, we come back to a holistic approach, where humans (idiosyncratic and individual) are treated as a whole.

PHARMACEUTICALS

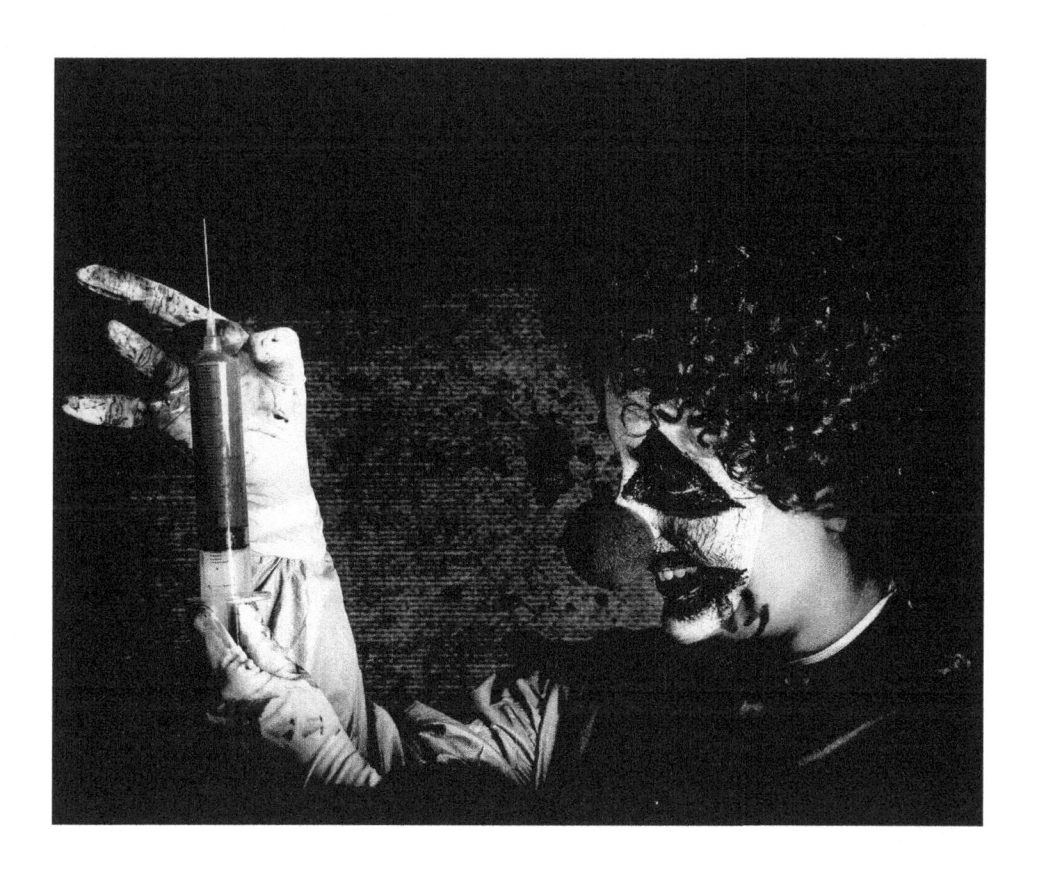

Why off labelling drug prescription is off its head

Off-label drug prescribing is now all the rage.

A recent report stated that Seroquel (Quetiapine) is now being used for sedation, depression and anxiety disorders.

It was originally used as a psychotic agent, along with Zyprexa and Risperdal, and was used mainly for poor old ladies (but not men) locked up in nursing homes — just before the makers of Soylent Green took over.

Old lady jaw melt

Many old ladies were also pumped full of bi-phosphonates to treat their osteoporosis when really they should have spent more time in the sun and never used sunscreen.

But an unfortunate side-effect of all this old lady bi-phosphonate-pumping was jaw necrosis, where the jaw just melted away.

Still, it stopped them from complaining.

Seroquel, Zyprexa and Risperdal are now used for treating children with ADHD and autism (also off-label).

To have children being assaulted by Ritalin and amphetamines is already bad enough, but adding the anti-psychotics is a direct attack on their still-evolving brain chemistry.

Somehow or other, doctors and psychiatrists have been convinced by Astra-Zeneca — a European/American conglomerate – to treat all these conditions they were never given approval for. Perhaps paid trips to very important conferences in Basle, Geneva and Disneyland may have something to do with it.

A crumbling insomniac

As well as crumbling in all directions, I have always had trouble sleeping.

I saw the local doctor and described the "restless legs" syndrome where I wrung my hands, twitched legs, rubbed my scalp and refused to nod off until 3 or 4am.

He mentioned that an off-label supply of Levodopa would be worth a try.

This was used for Parkinson's disease and seriously messed with your brain chemistry, and I thought my brain chemistry was pretty messy anyway. I tried it for three nights and then gave up — it didn't work and no-one could ever assess what harm it was doing.

Nudity cures my insomnia

I solved the problem of sleepless nights by going out into the garden with little or no clothes on (this is the horrifying part of the story), staying there until I started freezing and shivering and then went back to bed and slept.

This was cheaper and my brain chemistry stayed intact, though perhaps some minor changes would have helped. For example, brain chemistry alterations to help me believe that TV reality shows are real and to understand why we have a plethora of TV cooking shows in a nation that doesn't cook.

How to be the world's most inept drug pusher

I would go down as the most inept drug pusher of all time.

I was dubious from the start as I listened to all these medical experts sponsored by the drug companies. I accept now that most drug treatment is useless and may harm the patient.

Placebos have always been an embarrassment (the researchers ignore it and hope it goes away), and iatrogenic diseases, caused by diagnosis and drug treatment, have reached an alarming high.

No evidence statins increase longevity

Recently, the ABC's science program Catalyst ran two programmes about high cholesterol and the multi-billion-dollar drugs now used to treat it. The researchers (mostly American) simply said there was no evidence that taking the statins would increase longevity.

They also said that drug companies had falsified evidence and down-played side effects.

Fears of litigation, where lawyers employed by drug companies will prosecute any doctor who doesn't prescribe statins, means that Australian doctors always toe the line of least resistance.

Go back to animal fats

The American doctors suggest a good exercise regime, going back to animal fats, cutting out the expensive margarines — which taste like sludge – and reducing carbohydrates and junk food. Carbohydrate intake is currently recommended along with the statins and this seems to be a key factor in the staggering incidence of diabetes.

When I started in pharmacy, there were drug companies all over the world but they were more benign.

Burrows-Welcome in the UK and CSL in Australia were Government-run, not-for-profit entities and they poured all their money into research. There would be hundreds of drug companies, all with 3 or 4 lines each, but they have now amalgamated into 5 or 6 world-wide monoliths.

Big Pharma is truly evil, as is Big Tobacco, Big Oil, Big Supermarket Chains, Big Grog suppliers, Big Fracking and other giant, piratical corporations now squeezing the life out of this planet.

Doctors have always taken bribes

Doctors have always taken bribes. Pharmacists also, but on a much lower scale (I have the best collection of pens), and one rep would shout me lunch at the local pub. Those were the good old days when we shut for lunch for an hour.

Now, doctors and researchers get overseas trips and all expenses paid just to spruik the drug companies' latest propaganda.

Our politicians, off to the races, or weddings, or footy finals, or buying investment properties, could learn a thing or two.

Rotigotine: Another drug with weird and wonderful side effects

Rotigotine is a new drug for the treatment of Parkinsons disease and as with all drugs in this class, it plays with your brain chemistry.

It's in the form of a patch, applied every 24 hours, and without going into all the wondrous benefits (just marginally above the dreaded placebo), here is a list of side-effects:

Nausea, dizziness, dyskinesia (shaking), insomnia, vomiting and hallucinations, headache, somnolence and rashes at the site of application (itching, redness and burning).

Somnolence (sudden onset of sleep) should be quite a big worry. This is a "sleep attack" and can occur any time (some have been on rotigotine for about a year before the sleep attacks occur). It may occur when driving, using tools or operating machinery.

Side-effects, continued:

Increased libido, hypersexuality (this may be cancelled by sudden sleep attacks), compulsive behaviours, repetitive, meaningless actions ("Punding"—what a great word—could apply to watching TV cooking shows or driving on a freeway). Also included are binge-drinking and pathological gambling (hang on, has rotigotine been added to our water-supply?).

But wait, there's more:

Also, cardiac valve abnormality, blood-pressure changes, visual disturbances (retinal detachment), and melanoma and other skin cancers complete the list (but there may be more around the corner).

I was staggered at one of the "mabs" (mono-clonal antibodies) when I read about homicidal and suicidal tendencies (we hope that suicide comes first), but the side-effects of all new drugs seem weirder and weirder.

Sighed Effects - What drugs really do to you

Generic medicines have thrived in the last few years, and I have misgivings. For all the many failings of the big established drug companies (and there are many) at least they have researched and developed many of today's drugs – which can be viewed with dismay anyway, as I have outlined.

Generics don't change this – they simply offer the same dubious benefits as the original drugs, but cheaper. The generic companies don't do any research or development – they wait until patents expire and then produce and market a copy.

There are some pitfalls here: often the generic is not bio-equivalent to the original; they may have different fillers, preservatives etc., and could be quite different in their bio-availability, absorption rates, elimination rates and side-effects. They also come under a bewildering array of names, which gives rise to errors and confusion and there are many cases of doctors not realising that a patient is taking the same drug under two different names.

There is a psychological effect with many people relying on established brand names. The most notable one here is "Ventolin" with asthmatics depending on it heavily. If you are struggling for breath, Ventolin is rightly viewed as a life-saver, and the dependence is so strong that many will refuse cheaper generic versions.

In Australia, generics have been encouraged and promoted by Governments in an attempt to lower the overall health bills. This is done via the Pharmaceutical Benefits Scheme (PBS) where drugs are listed and subsidised. Listing on the PBS is supposed to be on purely medical grounds, but as in every Government/ Private partnership, there are many ways to pervert the system.

Drug company lobbyists exert influence on doctors and pharmacists with gifts, and sway politicians with electoral and financial help. The PBS pays pharmacists each month for the drugs dispensed and subsidised and the payment is based on wholesale drug prices paid by the pharmacy. This is where the generic companies (and pharmacists) have been ripping off the system for years.

To encourage pharmacists to use their particular brands, the companies offer huge discounts or bonus stock (or both), reducing the listed wholesale price to half or even less. This is not passed on to the PBS or to patients using generic drugs. It always amused me when I heard some pharmacists say to patients– "Would you like the cheaper generic Aussie brand", knowing that the pharmacist was reaping a financial benefit and that the "Aussie brand" was usually made in Mexico, South Africa or the Philippines.

PBS Fraud And Rorting

The PBS scheme is open to fraud and rorting with many pharmacies claiming for drugs they haven't actually dispensed. This requires signature forging which is seldom detected. I have some sympathy for many pharmacists who mildly exploit the system to help some of their poorer patients, or to redress the inevitable bureaucratic wrongs and anomalies that sometimes deprive them of a just income.

An Example Of Fraud

I will give just one example here out of many ways to exploit the PBS. I heard of a pharmacist being phoned by a local doctor, who asked if there was a way an elderly and poor pensioner could acquire a ventilating machine for his worsening asthma.

These machines cost up to $300 or $400 and are not subsidised. The pharmacist suggested the doctor could write a few rather pricy prescriptions for him, which he would "forget" to pick up. This would cover the cost of the machine, which was then donated to the patient, who never knew. On the face of it, this is fraud, but I believe it was simply a way of providing a vital service which should have been provided to him anyway.

Like all things, there are degrees of fraud, and there is no black and white. I know of many pharmacists who abuse the system for their own benefit, with some (the really blatant ones) getting caught eventually but most continuing on their merry way.

Trend To Huge, Discount Pharmacies Typical Of Greedy Consumerism

The trend nowadays is towards huge, discounting pharmacy chains, which I distrust because they are the real (and damaging) "drug-pushers", they are impersonal, they have a vested interest in generics and they are typical of the savage and ugly face of greed and consumerism.

On-Line Pharmacies Are Fraught With Danger

There is also a trend towards on-line pharmacies (quite often run by the same warehouse chains), which has been shown in the US to be fraught with danger. It has been stated that 95% of on-line pharmacies there are phonies— that is, they are actually based overseas. There is no guarantee of safety, with many of the drugs supplied being cheap copies with fake packaging, altered expiry dates and dubious sources. The FDA in America has closed many of them down but they change their name and immediately re-open.

Expiry Dates Are A Scare Campaign

On the issue of expiry dates, this has been a scare campaign and a rip-off also. The latest research shows that nearly all solid drugs stay stable and potent for decades after the nominal expiry date.

The whole system (which applies to food too, of course) has suited the big end of town manufacturers who have relied on timid Governments, fear of litigation (no wonder everyone hates lawyers), and propaganda, to induce fear into the general public about going a micro-second past the magic date.

I had a cavalier dis-regard for this system and, with the exception of aspirin, adrenalin and some anti-biotics, would provide expired drugs (at no cost) to friends and relatives (and even me).

Antibiotics are obviously useful and vital at times, yet their use will always alter natural (and beneficial) micro-organism levels, particularly bacteria and fungi.

There has always been disquiet about this wiping out of 'friendly' organisms, with thrush (candida — mostly in women) becoming wide-spread. There are now theories that the imbalances created by antibiotic therapy could even lead to autism in susceptible children.

Blood pressure

Blood pressure (BP) drug treatment is widely encouraged, but again these potent drugs are tailored to alter natural heart and kidney functions.

Blood pressure rises with age, but with good reason. All our systems deteriorate with age (shocking though that is) and start to falter.

Our hearts and kidneys compensate for this by using enzyme systems to slowly increase BP so that the faltering organs can get more oxygen.

The drugs are designed to either block this enzyme action, block calcium flow or act through the central nervous system, which achieves a drop in BP at the expense of drastic changes elsewhere.

Heart

The heart itself can be (and is) treated with all sorts of stimulants, again at the expense of naturally occurring changes.

Brain chemistry

Interfering with brain chemistry has become a ready fix.

Anti-depressants, anti-psychotics and anxiolytics are now routinely prescribed for all ages.

The dancing magic of these brain chemicals is really wondrous, ideally forming a balance with split-second timing by enzymes and enzyme destroyers.

Chemicals such as serotonin, nor-adrenalin, dopamine, GABA and others flit in and out of existence amid the infinite complexities of the neurons in the brain.

I consider drug treatment here to be crude, damaging and based on hope because no-one knows or understands why or how these drugs appear to sometimes work.

Why modern medicine is failing us all

I am appalled by the direction in which modern medicine is heading.

I've been retired from pharmacy for almost two years now and I still read up on the latest horrors.

The Western world is suffering epidemics of obesity, diabetes, heart disease, cancers, depression and arthritis.

Our children are increasingly unhealthy and many are born with ADHD, autism, dystrophies and other serious conditions. People demand instant fixes for all these things, so that's what they get.

Dabigatran is a new drug to replace Warfarin as a blood thinner. Warfarin is cheap but effective – with the disadvantage of requiring frequent blood tests. Dabigatran costs an arm and a leg (not literally), is equally effective BUT has been found to sometimes cause fatal hemorrhage.

And, to top it all off, there is no antidote.

Great work, fellas.

The monoclonal antibodies are now sweeping the world and if you are ordered a drug with a funny name ending in 'mab' run for your life.

These have been developed at great cost to treat the modern-day epidemics of so-called 'auto-immune' diseases – cancers, arthritis and other problems that can't be explained.

Using gene therapies and experimental mice, chickens and cows, the MABS are created and then spliced onto human antibodies. Costing thousands of dollars with each treatment, they are then used as immune-suppressants, the theory being they will prevent human rogue antibodies from causing disease.

Great theory, but stuffing around with the very complex human immune system is just stupid.

All kinds of side effects occur – opportunistic infections of course – which can be fatal, as well as far-reaching reactions body-wide.

I actually laughed out loud at a recent report on one of the latest MABS. It solemnly stated that one side-effect is "homicidal ideation".

Another side-effect is "suicidal ideation" – that is, you think killing yourself or someone else is a good idea.

Our medical system needs to acknowledge that we are all a collection of cells called 'life'.

Some cells are healthy, others defective.

Medicine needs to focus on prevention and improving environmental factors rather than treating modern-day 'life-style' disorders with dangerous, expensive and mostly useless drugs.

Poppin pills ain't curin' ills

I should say here that I have the greatest respect for many in our medical system. There are brilliant and concerned diagnostic doctors and skillful surgeons, but in general the system cranks and groans under enormous pressure, with many short-comings.

Doctors in general practice have little time to assess patients as individuals and usually know nothing of their lives, genetics or problems.

Fear Of Litigation

The fear of litigation explains why doctors are generally conservative and orthodox. Medical orthodoxy requires them to conform to all the latest drug treatments, pathology tests and a rigid scientific analysis of symptoms. There is little instinctive and skilled diagnosis, with constant referrals to specialists who know a hell of a lot about their very narrow fields, and nothing about the individual patient and holistic medicine.

All modern drug treatment is based on statistics and probability (and the profit motive). People vary widely in their responses to drugs, and this depends on age, genetics and naturally occurring and individualistic physiology (liver enzymes and the immune system are unique to each individual). For instance, people can be divided into 'fast metabolisers' and ' slow metabolisers', which is inherent and has a marked effect on drug absorption, distribution, break-down and excretion.

Another example is the effect of codeine. In most people, codeine is converted to morphine (which accounts for its analgesic effect and why some people become hooked on Panadeine Fort, Nurofen Plus etc.). In about 10% of people, the codeine remains unchanged and is thus less effective and sometimes quite disorientating.

The Placebo Effect

The varying metabolic responses to drug treatment are well known, but by unwritten consent (Noam Chomsky calls this "manufacturing consent"), they are ignored or treated as an "inconvenient truth". Another big (and embarrassing) factor in drug treatment is the placebo effect. This really rankles with the medical industry as all drugs have to be tested against placebo before they can be released.

The placebo statistics for effectiveness are always high (sometimes higher than the actual drug) and are simply ignored or down-played. The placebo will also induce just as many side –effects as the tested drug, but sometimes less. I have often thought of marketing a new "wonder drug", calling it Placebo Domingo, pushing it on to A Current Affair or Today Tonight and having confidence that it will measure up in effectiveness and not have any serious side-effects.

This placebo effect extends to cases of surgery where it can be quite embarrassing when 'pretend' surgery is just as effective as the real thing.

Overuse of Statin Class Drugs

Other worrying trends include the over-use of the statin class drugs for lowering cholesterol.

Higher than normal cholesterol levels have long been suggested as a risk factor in cardiovascular events. I have no doubt this is true, but that is all it is – a statistical risk factor, and again a natural physiological system is drastically altered.

Medical orthodoxy has decreed that everyone should lower their levels, which I find absurd. As always, individuals vary widely as to their natural levels since cholesterol is a natural, liver-produced compound essential as a building block for many hormones. Each person would have unique requirements and unique levels, depending on age, sex and genetics, but this is never considered. Instead, statins are routinely prescribed for just about everyone, with the latest propaganda (from drug company scientists) now recommending that they be given as a preventative against cardiovascular disease and cancer, even if the patient's cholesterol levels are low.

What is continuously played down or ignored completely are the sometimes serious side-effects of statins. These include mental confusion, insomnia and, more seriously, muscle pain, which can be relatively mild (myopathy) or severe to fatal (rhabdomyolysis – or muscle 'melt-down').

Most people taking statins can tolerate the liver enzyme- destroying action of the drug but any hint of muscle pain or soreness should be a clear signal to stop.

Treatment of gastric and oesophageal problems has also ballooned in recent times, with there being two theories. Excess acid – so the old antacids, bicarbonates and salts of magnesium, calcium and aluminium were used extensively until modern, high-potency antacids took over. Zantac, Tagamet and others prevailed for a while and then Losec, Nexium, and Somac stormed in. All these drastically reduce the hydrochloric acid naturally produced in the stomach to aid digestion so, again, a natural system was greatly reduced and modified.

The other theory was the presence of a bacterium – helicobacter - in some people's stomachs. The answer was an intense course of three potent antibiotics which, in my experience of people taking them, never seemed to work. But I have no doubt the antibiotics stuffed up their gastric systems even more. Helicobacter is so wide-spread in Western communities that I suspect it is only a problem when in imbalance — that is, antibiotic treatment, has killed off beneficial bacteria and allowed this one to flourish.

A parallel here is the treatment of giardia which is a naturally occurring protozoa in everyone's gut. Occasionally there is a rapid increase in its population, causing some mild diarrhoea. This is called giardiasis and is treated, of course, with antibiotics – which is madness since the overgrowth of giardia would have been due to antibiotic use or other environmental factors in the first place.

Possibly the worst and most damaging form of drug treatment nowadays is the use of immune-suppressants. The older drugs were bad enough (immune-suppressing chemotherapy for cancer and arthritis), but the new batches of "MABS" (mono-clonal antibodies) and "NIBS" (tyrosine kinase inhibitors) are frightening. They are designed to interfere with the body's natural immune system on the assumption that cancer, arthritis, MS, scleroderma, lupus and other modern scourges, are caused by auto-immune attacks—that is, the body's immune system is mistakenly attacking its own tissue. By their very nature, these drugs have serious side-effects, caused by reducing immunity all over the body, not just in the targeted areas. I have mentioned before that one of the latest "MABS' seriously listed suicidal ideation and homicidal ideation as side –effects, with the manufacturers possibly hoping that the suicidal bit occurs before the homicidal bit.

There would be many more examples of natural body systems being drastically changed by drugs, but the general theme is that modern drug treatment is badly flawed, based as it is on statistics, medical people fearful of litigation and the profit motive of the international drug cartels.

The fact that the most vulnerable people in our society, the youngest and the oldest, are now routinely over-treated with drugs, is worrying.

The elderly, mostly stashed away in nursing homes, are constantly drugged up. I suspect this is mostly for convenience and the economics of running a home. A large percentage of the drugs are anti-depressants, anti-psychotics, anxiolytics and sedatives. Laxatives and scabies lotions also get a good run and if the 'psyche' drugs don't turn the residents into zombies, this is soon fixed with massive doses of opiate analgesics.

I was recently given a guided tour of a pharmacy which catered only to nursing homes. This was in an industrial area, with the pharmacy occupying a huge, double-storeyed factory. I walked through a tiny, gloomy reception area and into a vision of Hell. Here were ranks of computers, automated drug-dispensing machines, huge reserves of drugs constantly being used or transferred (by conveyer belts), dozens of people rushing around making Webster Packs or checking the contents, storemen, accountants, and the occasional pharmacist.

I was told there were over 100 people employed here (with perhaps 3 or 4 pharmacists in all) serving dozens of nursing homes all over Melbourne. Apart from the alien concept (to me anyway) of this huge, impersonal organisation doling out enormous quantities of drugs to people they would never meet or know in any way, what also occurred to me was the old Charlton Heston film Soylent Green. This was a vision of a nightmare future where all the oldies, the maimed and the useless were periodically herded into a huge factory and fed Soylent Green.

I felt this drug factory was similar—instead of the oldies coming in for their Soylent Green, it was very kindly packed up and shipped out to them, courtesy of your friendly GP and drug supplier.

Equally vulnerable and exploited are the very young. This happens because of anxious parents, who are bombarded with drug company propaganda (treating teething, sniffles, mild temperatures, mild rashes, mild colic etc., as diseases, rather than childhood hiccups). Doctors are sucked into this over-treatment and concern, ordering sedatives, anti-depressants, stimulants (for ADHD) and even anti-psychotics. I dread what this neurological tampering is doing to the young, already under enormous environmental stress. Just some more premature recruits for the Soylent Green experience, I guess.

Why we crumble as we age and how modern medicine makes it worse

In my most recent article, I discussed the pitfalls of modern drugs and how they play havoc with our bodies. In this article, I will alert you to a few more examples of drug treatment interfering with our natural physiological healing processes.

Alarmingly, this is now the common approach to most of our long-term illnesses.

Crumbling People

Most of these chronic illnesses could be simply classified as aging— that is, major organs and systems "crumble" with age. Indeed, elderly patients admitted to ER in hospitals are referred to as "crumblers". They often have multiple organ failures and the hospital systems are hopelessly inadequate to cope with them.

It is estimated that there are 1500 deaths of "crumblers" per year due to excessive waiting times. The waiting occurs because specialists refuse to treat these inconvenient crumbling people, who actually need a GP trained in holistic medicine, who can examine, diagnose and treat their multiple disorders. This is recognised in the UK where there are many GPs employed in hospitals, but ignored in Australia.

We all age, deteriorate and turn into crumblers, but our system of ultra-specialisation (each specialist treating just one organ or system) is badly flawed.

Drug Treatment Anomalies

I first became aware of the anomalies of drug treatment when learning about the glycosides extracted from foxglove plants. This was called digitalis from which digoxin and digitoxin were isolated. Digoxin became the drug of choice for chronic heart failure (usually in the elderly) and I remember being perplexed when told the overall survival rate hardly changed. As the digoxin increased the heart output, the heart muscle itself swelled, became less efficient and sometimes induced heart-valve and pace-maker problems.

It didn't seem to matter as digoxin is still used today and the inconvenient truths about it ignored.

Attempts To Mimic Neuro-Transmitters

Another early development was based on the neuro-transmitters Acetylcholine and Cholinesterase. These flit in and out of existence in micro-seconds all over the body, allowing nerve impulses to pass into muscle receptors. They are thus integral to the successful function of all organisms and there were many attempts to develop drugs that mimicked or promoted their action. Nearly all of them failed because of the ephemeral and wide-spread nature of these neuro-transmitters, but a few are still being used (in desperation) to treat otherwise intractable problems like irritable bowel syndrome and gastric disorders.

The Bad News

The bad news is that the anti-cholinesterases took off in a big way with the development of hundreds of organo-phosphate pesticides and herbicides. Many of these were simply nasty and dangerous and were eventually banned, but some still persist. They do their killing by prolonging the action of acetylcholine, which then acts as a poison by paralysing natural communication systems.

The quantities drenching our farmlands, water tables and food chains (now including the ubiquitous Glyphosate or "Round-Up") are frightening and could explain many modern childhood neurological disorders.

Clouds Of Glyphosate

I shudder as I see pregnant women blithely walking through clouds of glyphosate being happily sprayed everywhere by jolly council workers, and home gardeners who believe the propaganda spruiked by the manufacturers. It is another madness to keep pouring this stuff into our already badly degraded environment, with the developing neurology of the un-born and the very young at intense risk.

An irony of all this is that the latest (desperate) attempts to treat Alzheimer's disease are expensive anti-cholinesterases, which may very well have contributed to the problem in the first place.

How our toxic environment is playing havoc with our children's health

Kas Thomas writes a thoughtful piece on environmental toxins (including the mercury-containing Thiomersol which is used in some vaccines) and their link to the staggering 50-fold rise in autism over the last three decades. The resident Midlifexpress pharma-shaman, Robert Gosstray, author of Pharmacy's Dirty Secrets, is angry that the increasingly toxic environment is compromising our children's biological health. Here's his take on the unfolding catastrophe:

The autism link to Thiomersol is valid. Mercury compounds, organic and inorganic, were big for quite a while — mostly for external use, but the mercury was absorbed through the skin anyway. They were used to treat eczema, lice, scabies, syphilis and other scrofulous disorders, and they were also used orally in tonics, powders, etc. It was thought that the Mercurous salts (Mercurous Chloride or Calomel) were less toxic than the Mercuric salts (and this was probably right), but they all did some damage, especially to children.

Calomel was a mercury compound used in teething powders and every second kid was regularly doped up. The result was an epidemic of Pink Disease — chronic mercury poisoning with all sorts of neurological and digestive problems.

We never learn.

Like any potentially dangerous (and wrong) practice, it is almost impossible to have it scientifically investigated, assessed and corrected. This is because one nasty factor in our environment is impossible to separate out from all the others.

I would have no doubt that Thiomersal causes damage (and autism) but it is working in conjunction with all the other environmental toxins we are afflicted with every second of our lives. Epidemiologists and other researchers would investigate Thiomersal in isolation and perhaps find no direct causal link. They haven't got the time, the interest or the money to investigate the nasty combinations of environmental contaminants we are drowning in.

THE GOLDEN AGE

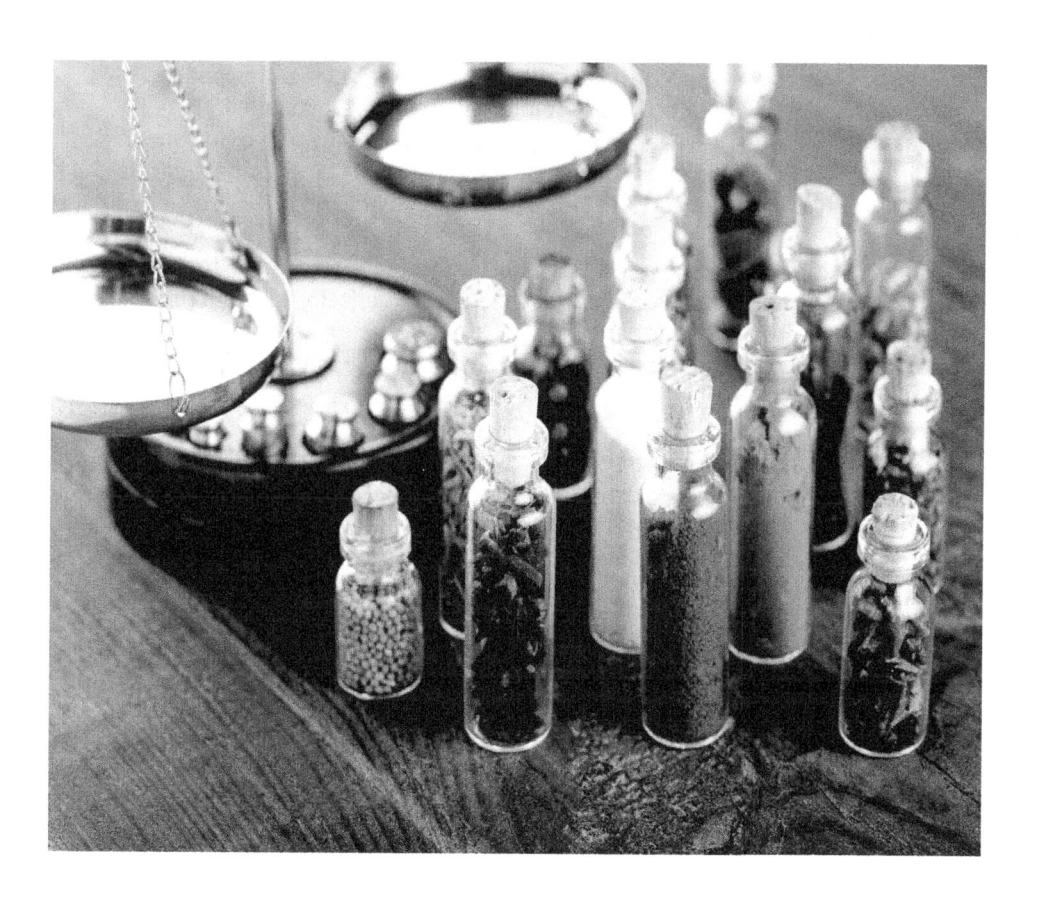

From Shaman to Pharman': Pharmacy's lost heritage

Pharmaceutical practices have changed considerably over the past fifty years. My first few years consisted of mixing, grinding with mortar and pestle, weighing, measuring, dissolving, heating, cooling, colouring, flavouring and depositing finished products into suitable bottles with appropriate, laboriously – typed directions. This was called extemporaneous dispensing and accounted for about 90 per cent of all prescriptions. The only ready-prepared items were a few antibiotics (penicillin and sulphonamides), barbiturates, thyroid extracts and a few others.

We made up an enormous range of mixtures, creams, ointments, lotions, liniments, eye, ear and nasal drops, suppositories, pills, pessaries, soaps, tinctures, spirits, emulsions, dusting powders, powders for internal use, elixirs, gels, inhalations, linctuses (lincti?) pastes and even injections. These were mostly based on Formularies – the British Pharmacopeia (and Codex), and the APF (Australian Pharmaceutical Formulary),with some American and European formulae thrown in.

These preparations had been passed down through the ages, based on herbal, animal and mineral sources. I believe some of them were just as effective or even more so, than current modern drug treatment. They were also less expensive and had few side-effects. There was little treatment for cardiovascular ailments, and none at all for cancer except morphine.

This extemporaneous system worked well, with doctors and pharmacists having knowledge and being trained, to prescribe and dispense respectively (and respectfully). It obviously took more time to dispense these compounds, and was probably the origin of – "that will be about 20 minutes", said to each patient. We shortened much of the dispensing time by making up pre-prepared stock solutions and concentrates.

I enjoyed the extemporaneous system, getting great satisfaction and knowledge from pharmacology, botany, material medica, pharmacognosy (drugs extracted from plant sources), drugs from mineral and animal sources, organic chemistry, physics and forensics. We were educated on incompatibilities (no- not Tom Cruise and Katie), especially when making up emulsions and creams—with the wrong combinations, these would "crack", separating into gooey oily and watery messes – hastily dumped into the nearest bin.

The dispensing techniques used the apothecary system of weights and measures when I started, so we measured in grains, drachms, ounces, minims, fluid drachms and ounces, and occasionally pints, pounds, quarts and gallons (for bulk dispensing and hypochondriacs). Doses of liquids were given as teaspoons or tablespoons, and prescriptions were scrawled out by doctors in a mixture of old Latin, arcane abbreviations and symbols, and occasionally, even modern English.

Some of the writing was truly terrible but we managed to decipher most of it. One memorable scrawl from my early days was a script for "Pulv. ABT". I knew "pulv" was

Latin for "powder" but the "ABT" had me tossed - no such thing in any formulary I knew. I rang the doctor who just said, "Give him Any Bloody Thing- he's a hypochondriac".

This apothecary system changed later into the metric system which is probably more logical and consistent, but didn't have the same charm. All our dispensing was based on centuries – old methods of combining, blending and compounding various naturally occurring substances which were standardised and purified.

These formulae and techniques were based on old, sometimes pre-historic, hunter-gatherer societies who had learnt - by bitter experience - which plants were safe and useful. Shamans, medicine men (and women) and community leaders passed this knowledge on to succeeding generations, eventually forming the basis of European medical practice right up to recent times. It is only in the last 50 years or so that this system has been almost totally replaced by modern potent drugs, big Government and giant multi-national drug cartels.

Up until the late 1950s, pharmacists mixed 90 per cent of their medicines on site (called extemporaneous dispensing). Nowadays, everything is pre-packed and there is virtually no extemporaneous dispensing. I regret this up to a point - there was a certain charm, elegance and skill in the dispensing methods which are now totally lost. Modern pharmacies have even lost their distinctive smell as all the vast array of natural and exotic substances, all leaching their subtle odours into the air, were replaced by a sterile array of packaged pills and tablets.

Since we had large stocks of poisons and narcotics, we also had very tight controls on sales and recording. We were governed by laws from various Medical Acts, Pharmacy Acts and Poisons Acts, with multitudes of Government and semi-Government agencies all regularly sending out inspectors to check on us. I always made sure that everything balanced in regard to narcotics—we had to record everything exactly, which was only right.

However, working on the assumption that inspectors were appointed and paid to inspect and detect faults, errors or carelessness, I always made sure there were a few minor discrepancies here and there. These were duly found and reported on, and I gave the inspector a nice cup of tea, while nodding agreeably to his helpful suggestions of how I could be more efficient. Everyone was happy- he could report to his superiors about the faults he had found and I would receive a gentle reprimand or advice on how to conduct myself properly.

Forensic pharmacy relating to the laws surrounding the manufacture, selling, storage and recording of poisons, narcotics and potent drugs, was a large and interesting part of pharmacy practice. I abided by the majority of the laws but broke a few when it was in the interests of our patients. The various poisons and drugs were classified into eight schedules. Dangerous poisons were sch.1, prescription only drugs were sch.4 and narcotics were sch.8.

I was fascinated by all the ancient schedule 1 poisons. If we sold any, we had to enter the details in a poisons book. The sales included Pitts Wheat, a strychnine based grain for foxes, rats and mice, Edison's Exterminator (starring Arnold Schwarzenegger) for ants, flies, earwigs, fleas and other vermin, tartar emetic containing antimony for ants, errant husbands (thank you Agatha Christie) and making you vomit, arsenic, mercury and lead salts, cyanides, corrosive acids and alkalis, and many plant-based poisons from belladonna, aconite, foxglove, oleander and castor-oil plants.

The regulations on what was dangerous changed with bewildering speed at times, an example being Selsun shampoo which was listed in schedule 1. This meant everyone with dandruff had to sign the poisons book, giving reasons for purchase. It contained selenium which had been part of yet another Agatha Christie plot involving cheating husbands and murderous wives, but, as always, our authorities over-reacted, fearing an Australian outbreak of shampoo-based homicides. Things like Shelltox pest strips and Lawson's Bronchitis mixture were also on sch.1 for a while, which was equally ridiculous and comical.

From the 1960's onwards, all this quaint, charming, and slow-paced way of life changed rapidly, as drug companies and Government researchers took over by developing thousands of new, expensive compounds in an attempt to guarantee perfect health for everyone (if they had money). That will be my next daring treatise on our drugged-out society.

A modern alchemist recalls the golden years of pharmacy

Following on from my less than complimentary comments on modern-day medical practices and the drugs they prescribe, here is a description of pharmacy as I first practised it.

I qualified in 1961 after being apprenticed for 4 years. I was following in the footsteps of all those ancient apothecaries who had been seeking to convert base metals into gold and to discover the Elixir of Youth. In breaking news (remember, you heard it here first), I did none of these things and concentrated on dispensing, compounding, formulating and occasionally procrastinating.

More breaking news: I now confess — I did convert all that dross to gold and I did find the Elixir of Youth, but I selfishly kept it all to myself. If you see an extremely good looking and youthful bloke paying for his Wheaties with small nuggets of gold, that's me.

I spent my days making exotic preparations based on centuries of research

My days were spent making up huge ranges of preparations which we had all been well trained for at the Pharmacy College and in apprenticeship. These preparations were all based on hundreds of years of research and experience in using mostly botanical extracts and they were valid and effective for their time, with the big advantage of not having the enormous range of side-effects common to modern drugs.

It was labour intensive, time consuming and inexpensive as we made up eye drops, ear drops, nasal drops, inhalations, mixtures, creams, ointments, emulsions, lotions, liniments, pills, suppositories, douches, pessaries, powders, pastes, syrups, and many other compounds. It was necessary to learn about all types of solvents, solubilities of substances in these solvents, incompatibilities (where some substances would interact), dosages for adults, children and babies, as well as weights and measures (I first used the apothecary system of grains, drams, ounces, minims, fluid ounces and then changed to the metric grammes and millilitres).

Exotic poisons

I was fascinated by the huge collections and varieties of substances we used. Poisons of all kinds were in constant use, with the trick being able to use them in appropriate dosages and circumstances. We had stocks of all the heavy metals and their salts — Mercury, Lead, Arsenic, Copper, Zinc, Antimony and Iron — as well as stocks of organic poisons such as strychnine, cyanides and aconite.

Deadliest poison in the universe

We had some aconitine, the active alkaloid of Aconite (or wolf's bane) and God knows why we had it. Aconitine is probably the deadliest poison in the universe, suited only for use by Russian KBG agents who stab people with umbrella tips.

More exotic poisons

We had green, white and blue vitriols — Sulphates of Iron, Zinc and Copper which had been put to great use by Lucrezia Borgia in Medieval times. The Belladonna and Digitalis alkaloids were also very potent, as well as more obscure things like Cantharides — the dried powder obtained from crushing beetles. Called 'Spanish Fly', it was used as an aphrodisiac but would have killed more men than it helped.

Other exotic poisons were Oil of Tansy, Oil of Mirbane and Ricin (obtained from castor oil seeds and another favourite umbrella-tip poison). A good example of a balanced use of poisons in small doses, was QES tablets. As I have previously mentioned, QES was the only effective abortion agent available for many years, and the combination of Quinine, Ergot and Strychnine — all poisons — worked well in the small doses given.

Vale the pharmacy of old

Previously, I described pharmacy as I first practised it fifty years ago. It was more wholistic (and much more aromatic) in those days because we used whole plant extracts to produce a gentler, less toxic pharmaceutical bounty than we have today. Here are a few more strange and exotic lotions and tinctures I made in that long-gone era.

Volatile and fixed oils — an aromatic heaven

Another big group of substances we used to make medicines were volatile and fixed oils. The volatile oils were derived from plants and were very aromatic, which contributed greatly to the characteristic smell of old pharmacies (lavender, orange, lemon, citronella, rose, rosemary, cardamom, Siberian fir, bergamot, cajuput, dill, caraway, aniseed, juniper, mustard, eucalyptus, eucalyptol, almond, cedar, orange-flower, cinnamon, and raspberry).

There were few unpleasant smells – several sulphides and some solvents – and smell played a big part in identifying benign and not-so-benign agents. We used many solvents — ethanol, methanol, chloroform, acetone, ether, propyl alcohol, amyl acetate (smelled like bananas), acetaldehyde, benzene, fixed oils (olive, peanut, castor oil) and good old tap water. We were supposed to use sterile or distilled water but I always thought if it was good enough to drink, it was good enough to use in medicines.

Other exotica

Other substances included oxymels (honeys), paraffins (liquid, hard and soft), wool fat and lanoline, cocoa butter, beeswax, emulsifying agents, syrups and other sweeteners, liquorice, huge ranges of dyes and ancient galenicals (gelsem, senega, gentian, lobelia, strammonium, rhubarb, ginger, colchicum, peppermint, camphor, menthol, thymol, resorcinol, phenol, creosote, coal tars of many varieties, strong acids such as Sulphuric, Hydrochloric, Nitric, Phosphoric, Acetic, Hydrobromic and alkalis such as Caustic Soda and Strong Ammonia).

Similar to cooking, there was a certain amount of satisfaction in creating creams, mixtures and other compounds, with smoothness, colour and smell all being important. We had a huge range of dyes and aromatic agents to achieve this and I have to admit to occasionally being tempted to taste a particularly enticing cream (this was weird and probably illegal).

We used pure plant extracts

What we were practising was somewhat holistic in approach since we used pure plant extracts such as opium, belladonna, cannabis, ergot, digitalis, colchicum, cinchona, senega, gentian and many others. These contained varying amounts of active alkaloids, glycosides, tannins, alcohols, and esters which had medicinal effects. For instance, opium tincture and camphorated tincture of opium contained morphine, papaverine, noscapine and codeine.

These tinctures were prescribed for coughs, pain and sedation (in combination with kaolin to treat diarrhoea and in combination with senega extract and ammonium bicarbonate to treat coughs).

The ridiculous panic over Senega and Ammonia cough mixture

The saga of Senaga & Ammonia cough mixture is illustrative of panicky legislators conniving with the medical professions to fight the scourge of little old ladies with coughs becoming opium fiends. This wonderfully effective cough expectorant was neutered by replacing camphorated tincture of opium with camphor spirit. From then on, it was mass produced and distributed by drug companies who also removed chloroform from the formula. Liquorice extract and chloroform water had been used for ages to sweeten and preserve many mixtures and was particularly effective in masking the bitterness and sharpness of the senega, ammonium bicarbonate and the opium. The senaga and ammonia mixture had been reduced to a pale and less effective blandness.

Chloroform was also banned (along with morphine tincture) when Chlorodyne was banned. This was a brilliant combination of chloroform and morphine, which would instantly correct any case of diarrhoea with just a few drops dosage.

Another great favourite

Another great old favourite was "Four Three-penn'ths" which consisted of equal parts opium tincture (laudanum), camphorated opium tincture (paregoric), aniseed spirit and peppermint spirit. Again, with just a few drops dosage, it was used for a wide range of gastric problems (and a sedative and an anti-depressant). The notorious and vicious little old ladies loved this old favourite which must have originally cost them a whole shilling to buy.

Another very good cough mixture was Ipecac and Squill, a mixture of two tinctures- ipecacuanha (which in higher dosage is a very effective emetic) and Scillae (in higher doses a cardio-toxin). In small and balanced doses, flavoured with honey (oxymel), this was safe even for infants.

Bromides were often prescribed to lower the sex drive of men. They were used extensively in the First World War, being doled out to soldiers in order to take their minds off sex and concentrate on slaughtering people instead. The only other treatment doled out by army doctors was Gentian Violet which was splashed over everything from tinea to syphilis.

My next post will examine other well-established, cheap and effective concoctions from the past and the relentless and destructive inroads modern drug companies have made into the holistic pharmacy of old.

The aromatic heaven of the pharmacy of old

The aromatic pharmacy of old is gone and it's been replaced by an army of bland, potent and expensive medications with sterile names and lurid plastic packaging.

The holistic nature of all the compounds I mixed didn't occur to me at the time, but I now think this was their main benefit. By using complete plant extracts instead of the isolated active principles (which became a tidal wave of isolation and specialisation over the years), much was achieved with something lost when only the active ingredient was used. For example, using Morphine instead of the Opium extracts increased addiction rates and side-effects.

This reductionism has carried through to modern drug practice, which I feel is on the wrong track.

These great compounded mixtures all had an equivalence in tablet form, which was more convenient but lost the holistic appeal of the liquid form. APC mixture was a wonderful, finely balanced treatment for all kinds of pain, consisting of Aspirin, Phenacetin and Caffeine, flavoured with Orange Syrup and Chloroform water with the aspirin and phenacetin being suspended (they were insoluble in most solvents) by a gum called Tragacanth. It was a smooth and well-tolerated preparation suitable for all ages, and had a rapid onset of action.

The APC tablets were nowhere near as effective but they were convenient. This formula was frowned upon, with the phenacetin being replaced by Paracetamol, a much less effective pain-killer. The whole range of APC preparations, especially the commercially produced ones – Aspro, Bex, Vincents (powders and tablets) and others were gulped down by anxious and desperate housewives all over the world, with some reports of kidney damage. This was enough for another ban, which induced them to switch to Paracetamol (liver damage), ibuprofen (cardiovascular and gastric problems), Valium (even more addictive) and codeine (addictive and constipating).

Trend is to ban cheap older drugs and replace with expensive drugs

It is probably just coincidence (haw!) but it seems that the prevailing trend is to ban cheap and effective older drugs and replace them with expensive and more damaging drugs that are heavily promoted to doctors by the drug companies. This applies to amphetamines, opiates, cannabis and other groups which have all been banned.

Our moral guardians ban the wrong things

Our enlightened moral guardians also delight in banning books, plays, art and films. This censorious and over-protective attitude sits strangely with the reluctance to tackle the damage caused by alcohol, pornography, poor quality and violent TV shows, drugs in sports, family violence, religious bigots, racism and poverty.

This reluctance is not all that strange since it is far easier to attack and ban the so-called vices of the underprivileged — street drugs, grog, gambling, tobacco and sex. It is much harder to attack anyone or any group who can afford teams of lawyers. We often hear of police "swooping" on marijuana crops, crystal meth labs, bikie gangs, squatters, environmental activists and street demonstrators. They never "swoop" on crooked developers and the politicians in their pockets, or greedy and reckless bankers, or monolithic retail monopolies, or the oil and mining industries with their shameful history of exploitation and environmental damage.

If the medical, legal and political establishments were fair-dinkum, they would ban or clamp down on advertising.

Everyone knows that we (and particularly the younger generations) are being damaged by junk food, alcohol, sugary drinks, and a polluted and degraded environment. The level of advertising has reached enormous and intrusive levels, and this includes the simplistic and somewhat obscene ads for mining companies, whereby the miners are depicted as benevolent employers of indigenous people, in complete harmony with the environment and only doing this noble and selfless job for the benefit of all Australians.

The 'trickle-down' effect is a fiction.

These mining magnates pay little or no tax as they rapaciously gouge out as much as they can before it all runs out. A disturbing fact now emerging about the over-fed, underactive lifestyles of modern children in Western societies is that, for the first time, the coming generation will have a shorter life-span than the previous one. This should set off alarm bells, but the economic and environmental dead-end we have created, will mean the same destructive patterns will continue.

I enjoyed the complexities of old style compounding pharmacy,

I took great pride in producing safe, cheap and effective preparations from a wide range of materials, all done to time-tested formulae and catering to a wide range of people.

The people were the best part– unpretentious, obliging and of infinite character. One lady always asked us for "Angel-Jesus" balm, instead of "Analgesic Balm", one bloke would always rush back in saying " I forgot to get my memory pills and could I have some Black-jack too?" (an opium-containing cough mixture).

Another rather stupid customer would buy things and then always say,"I'm my father's son – do I get a discount?" One pimply-faced kid would always come in on Saturday mornings with a prescription for Sulphurated Potash Lotion. I hated making this — you had to crush up the potash with a mortar and pestle, liberating great clouds of "rotten-egg" gas and then take a few hours to dissolve it. No sweet aromatic smells on those days (and he stayed spotty anyway).

A notorious whinger brought in a prescription one day for "Pulv ABT". I scratched my head as I had never heard of this antacid preparation and it was in no reference book that I knew of. Reluctantly (taking some pride in always accurately interpreting any written prescription), I rang the doctor who just snorted –"It is Pulv Any Bloody Thing- he is a raging hypochondriac". I mixed up some bicarb, sugar and starch.

The decline in this form of compounding and dispensing was mainly caused by economic factors.

Medically, I would still have great faith in the time-tested formulae we used, but of course, there was no money in it for the big drug companies and therefore no promotion. Indeed their propaganda over the years has denigrated the old ways and promoted high-tech and expensive cure-alls for an increasingly self-obsessed and worried populace.

I regret the passing of these dispensing practices and the loss of the associated skills and knowledge, but realise it was of another much slower and less frantic time with people just happy to get by, without being obsessed with staying young and healthy forever.

Why I'm uneasy about our magic fix society

I am uneasy about the way our stress-ridden society now depends on a 'magic fix' for everything, which is catered for by a conservative and orthodox medical system.

Increasingly over the years, I have swung around to an holistic, instinctive approach for treating human ailments, and a preference for preventative medicine, rather than therapeutic.

As the avalanche of potent, ready-prepared drugs took over in my pharmacy, I gained a minor reputation for preserving many of the old stocks of galenicals, which encouraged some doctors and other pharmacists to send people to me for the old formulas.

I carried this through right up to the time I retired two years ago, but with increasing difficulty as old customers died (not my fault!) and stocks of the old substances gradually dwindled.

Growing unease

My growing unease with modern drug treatment is based on a consideration of the human body's complexity.

We are not just a collection of cells, organs and systems that modern treatment targets and alters (sometimes for the worse).

The body consists of finely balanced cells all working to maintain a healthy equilibrium in all our major systems.

It also consists of countless micro-organisms such as bacteria, viruses, fungi, protozoa, mites, and annelids (worms, don't shudder).
And it may surprise you to know there are more bacteria than human cells in a body.

State of harmony

All these organisms live in a state of harmony and usefulness unless disturbed.

Disturbances can arise from anatomical or physiological defects – some inherited or congenital.

Body disturbances also occur with allergies, infections from external pathogenic micro-organisms, poisoning, excesses in eating and drinking or any of our present-day temptations, accidents or just bad luck.

The disturbances produce imbalances in the finely-tuned and complex bodily systems.

Drug treatment seeks to correct these imbalances, and has some degree of success.

Modern medical practice, however, has neither the time, the money or (sadly) the interest, to consider each person as an individual, with perhaps idiosyncratic and individual body systems, functions, personalities and responses to potent drugs.

Here are some examples of how drug treatment affects bodily systems and functions:

Antibiotics

Antibiotics are obviously useful and vital at times, yet their use will always alter natural (and beneficial) micro-organism levels, particularly bacteria and fungi.

There has always been disquiet about this wiping out of 'friendly' organisms, with thrush (candida — mostly in women) becoming wide-spread. There are now theories that the imbalances created by antibiotic therapy could even lead to autism in susceptible children.

Blood pressure

Blood pressure (BP) drug treatment is widely encouraged, but again these potent drugs are tailored to alter natural heart and kidney functions.

Blood pressure rises with age, but with good reason. All our systems deteriorate with age (shocking though that is) and start to falter.

Our hearts and kidneys compensate for this by using enzyme systems to slowly increase BP so that the faltering organs can get more oxygen.

The drugs are designed to either block this enzyme action, block calcium flow or act through the central nervous system, which achieves a drop in BP at the expense of drastic changes elsewhere.

Heart

The heart itself can be (and is) treated with all sorts of stimulants, again at the expense of naturally occurring changes.

Brain chemistry

Interfering with brain chemistry has become a ready fix.

Anti-depressants, anti-psychotics and anxiolytics are now routinely prescribed for all ages.

The dancing magic of these brain chemicals is really wondrous, ideally forming a balance with split-second timing by enzymes and enzyme destroyers.

Chemicals such as serotonin, nor-adrenalin, dopamine, GABA and others flit in and out of existence amid the infinite complexities of the neurons in the brain.

I consider drug treatment here to be crude, damaging and based on hope because no-one knows or understands why or how these drugs appear to sometimes work.

Peak advertising of harmful products is here

Advertising of harmful substances has reached a peak

I have tackled this problem before, but the continuing promotion of grog, cigarettes, good dope, bad dope, gambling, medicines fake and real, and gigantic, sterilised sporting events played by rich robots have reached a peak.

Advertising has reached a screaming crescendo. Newspapers, TV, radio, and every sporting event now blatantly promote all these harmful influences on our society.

Karl Marx said that religion is the opium of the people and now all these things have replaced it.

I would like to see our economy-driven nightmare of a world switch over to a more reflective and considerate style.

This would mean no advertising of harmful products.

Recently, I went to see a movie and was assailed, assaulted and tortured by 45 minutes of ads for junk food, grog, gambling, cars and other consumer goods that no-one wanted, all at 155 decibels.

By the time the movie started, I just wanted to get out of there. (It was American Hustle—too long, too American, too contrived, but good acting.)

Peak sport advertising

Advertising is now so tied up with big sports events that everything is a brand.

Last year's Essendon Football Club peptide scandal is a good example.

We have the Essendon Football Club "brand" where corrupt pseudo-scientists assured gullible coaching staff that peptides were essential just to keep up with other teams. The AFL "brand" then defended the Essendon "brand", because they would lose too much money.

Peptides, by the way, are naturally occurring substances in the human body, involved with all organs (including Endorphin, the natural pain-killer).

It was truly awful that the peptide scandal at Essendon football club found no-one at fault.

Peptides have been around for a few years , mostly useless, but sometimes with a few amphetamine-like substances.

They were impossible to ban, since they varied in one or two molecules which altered their nomenclature.

Some doctors recommend taking peptides (for young athletes) and also give them steroid and testosterone injections. This is a short-sighted fix which does tremendous harm.

To mess around with this system is on a par with prescription drugs doing the same.

Peak vitamin and mineral advertising

And then we have the crass ads for vitamins and minerals that now appear in newspapers two or three times a week.
In the good old days, the only vitamin supplement was Vitamin B group Fort. This ultimately was turned into Myadec and Pluravit, with the addition of trace elements, metallic salts and amino acids.

These were harmless and occasionally did some good for a nutrition-deficient person, but mostly (90% or more), they were excreted in urine, flushed down the toilet and ended up in fish.

Peak advertisers love the People Who Want To Live Forever

But now we have weird and wonderful products from all over the world— advertise these (with no evidence of their value), and The People Who Want To Live Forever (TPWWTLF) spend huge amounts of money on Krill Oil, Shark cartilage, seaweed, green-lipped mussels, monkey glands, horns and antlers from various, rather unfortunate animals— it's a pity there is no market for flies, mosquitos, and cane toads.

You repeat a lie often enough and TPWWTLF will not only vote for you, but also waste their money on this rubbish.
Just about all modern ailments are based on poor sanitation, poor nutrition, poor drinking water, pollutants in food and air and, of course, genetics.

No-one (not even TPWWTLF) can dodge this.

Preventing all these evil influences on our lives (except for the genetics, but researchers are now pouring money into how to get better antecedents), should be the way to go, but there is no money in it.

Peak advertising rules all. What is good for KFC, Hungry Jacks, Maccas, Coke, getting drunk and violent and gambling until you are broke, must be good for us and the economy.

Economic Growth Model Infiltrates Health Care

In line with the global trend towards economic growth and "bigger is better", it is no surprise that Australian institutions have tagged along. Doctors and medical centres have been taken over by faceless groups of accountants, nursing homes the same (many owned by "Bluescope"), veterinarians (owned by Greencross) and (heaven forbid), pharmacies (Chemists Warehouse/My Chemist franchises). There is a very real possibility that many pharmacies will soon be swallowed up by Coles and Woolworths.

Being a grumpy old fogey, I don't like any of this but realise it is the price we pay for modern society's fixation with consumerism, cheaper prices and materialistic "success".

Present Day Medical Practice

A striking example of present-day medical practice happened when a surgery near my place of employment began stocking antibiotics, vaccines and other products. The doctor would not only prescribe these but also supply them, saying, " It will be cheaper here than at a pharmacy."

There has been a long history, achieved by consensus and ethics, of doctors and pharmacists not encroaching on each other's territory, and I felt this was a clear case of conflict of interest. This grated with my own ethics (yes – I do have some), so I wrote to the Medical Board, the Pharmacy Board and other bodies. They all ignored me except the Medical Board, who then investigated.

After two years, they were still investigating but finally reached a decision. They told me they had no jurisdiction to prevent this, though admitting it violated ethical standards, and that the doctors had said that their accountants had told them they needed to increase their turnover. I wrote back, saying, "Don't we all?", thanked them for nothing and forgot all about it.

Some practices also have very cosy arrangements (kick-backs) with pathology companies which have grown enormously in recent times due to doctors not having the time or skill to diagnose (and the fear of litigation if they don't order multiple tests for everyone). If there was no bulk-billing by Medicare and patients had to pay for this over-servicing, there would be a dramatic fall in the number of tests.

Horror Drug Treatments In Modern Medical Practice

Getting back to medical practice and drug treatment, here are some more things to consider:

Anti-inflammatories are routinely prescribed and dispensed for every minor muscle strain and in back pain. They are designed to reduce inflammation and this they do very well. The fact that this directly interferes with (and stops) the natural healing system, is ignored. When there is nerve or muscle damage anywhere in the body, fluid, enzymes and proteins called prostaglandins are rushed to the site, where they naturally cause swelling. This swelling is a sign of the healing process, so to artificially reduce or remove it, is madness.

Allied to the over-use of these drugs is the high incidence of side-effects. A drug called

"Vioxx" was banned a few years ago because of serious cardiovascular problems. Not mentioned is that there are still drugs on the market that are just as bad. Diclofenac (which can be sold without a prescription) has recently been found to have the same or worse side-effect profile as Vioxx, and ALL anti-inflammatories can cause gastric bleeding. When used in conjunction with anti-hypertensives and diuretics, they can cause kidney failure. Perhaps we should all stick exclusively to RICE – Rest, Ice, Compression and Elevation— and then do your own physiotherapy.

A report from America has mentioned that there is currently no research being done in developing new psychiatric drugs. Anti-depressants, anti-psychotics and anxiolytics all mess around with brain chemistry (often to the detriment of the patient), but the drug companies have decided there is no more money to be made in this field and have reverted to their favourite "cash-cows"— cancer, cardiovascular disorders and auto-immune diseases. These dominate our aging, health-obsessed and affluent populations, so that is where the money goes.

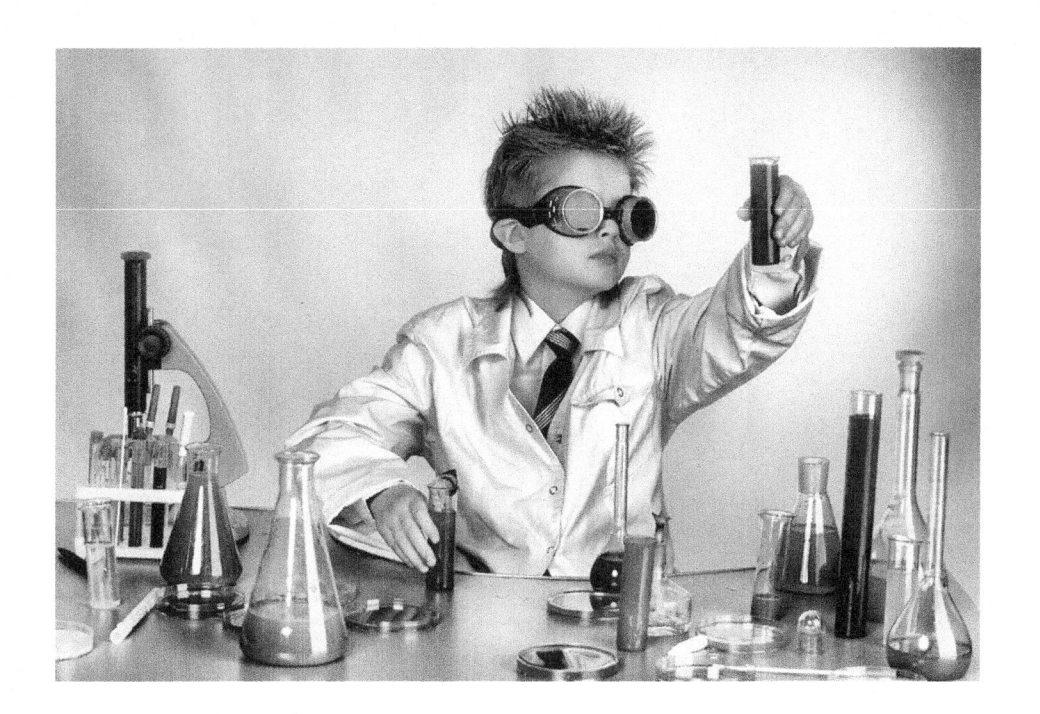

Robert Gosstray is a retired pharmacist who writes regularly for Midlifexpress. He's had enough of dodgy drug companies, mainstream malarkey and the dire eco/financial/social predicament engulfing our species. This zero-tolerance codex is a compilation of popular posts where he explores life, death, addiction (legal and illegal), the inane War on Drugs, modern (but still medieval) cancer treatment, ageing, and our desperate, futile desire to live forever.

Made in the USA
Monee, IL
17 June 2021